PENGUIN BOOKS
THE ART AND SCIENCE OF PEAK PERFORMANCE

John Aguilar is an award-winning serial entrepreneur, best-selling author, sprints and decathlon champion, and lifelong athlete. As a 'method producer', he has seamlessly integrated his business reality show *The Final Pitch* and documentary series *Methods to Greatness* to his own life, inspiring people to take their own entrepreneurial and wellness journeys. He is also the author of the best-selling books *The Art and Science of the Pitch: A Playbook for Pitching to Partners, Investors, and Reality TV Shows* and *Methods to Greatness: Lessons of the Mind, Body, and Soul from Asia's Top Entrepreneurs, Athletes and Icons*.

John is a seasoned business and motivational keynote speaker, having given talks on his experiences as an entrepreneur, content producer, pitching expert, innovation thinker, and peak performer. John holds an undergraduate degree in Science Psychology from Ateneo de Manila University, a master's in Entrepreneurship from the Ateneo de Manila Graduate School of Business and is an alum of Singularity University in Silicon Valley. He lives in Manila with his wife and three children

The Art and Science of Peak Performance

A Personal Journey to Enhance
Your Mind, Optimize Your Body,
and Live a Full Life

John Aguilar

PENGUIN BOOKS

An imprint of Penguin Random House

PENGUIN BOOKS

Penguin Books is an imprint of the Penguin Random House group of companies
whose addresses can be found at global.penguinrandomhouse.com

Published by Penguin Random House SEA Pte Ltd
40 Penjuru Lane, #03-12, Block 2
Singapore 609216

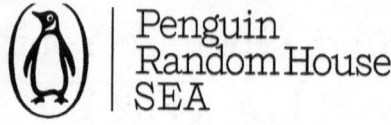

Penguin
Random House
SEA

First published in Penguin Books by Penguin Random House SEA 2025

The views and opinions expressed in this book are the author's own and the
facts are as reported by him which have been verified to the extent possible,
and the publishers are not in any way liable for the same.

ISBN 9789815233148

Typeset in Garamond by MAP Systems, Bengaluru, India

www.penguin.sg

For my father Dave and my son David,
May we make many more memories to remember.

Contents

Introduction

My wife always jokes about the fact that she hates my body.

That's because no matter what I eat, for some consistent (and unfair, in her mind) reason, I never seem to gain weight. I can almost tell like clockwork what I'll weigh every morning when I step on our digital weighing scale. But that's not the thing that she finds irritating. Because believe it or not, I actually lose weight when I stop exercising.

The compounding effect of some form of training or exercise integrated into my everyday for the past thirty-five years has moulded my body into a fat and calorie burning machine. Even at forty-six, as of this book's writing, my body, according to the body composition analyzer, has the metabolic age of a thirty-one-year-old, fifteen years younger than my chronological age. When I don't get to exercise, my body doesn't crave the calories I would normally need to sustain my activities, thereby decreasing my appetite and making me lose weight.

Except for the lack of a full head of hair, I've also been told that I don't look too far off from what I looked like when I was in my twenties. Vanity is definitely a contributing factor to this, as I have always wanted to look and feel good every time I look in the mirror.

I've also started training and competing again, more than two decades after retiring from track and field. I've held a number of high school and collegiate records in sprints, pole vaults, and the gruelling ten-event decathlon. I never really made it to the Philippine national team as I decided to retire early and pursue a career, so the sports thing had taken a back seat until now.

One would easily assume that everything under the hood is working optimally, but that's unfortunately not the case. I have twice the normal levels of LDL or 'bad' cholesterol no matter how disciplined I am with my lifestyle. This paradox exists in various forms in some aspects of my life. My sleep could come like clockwork one night and be totally off the next because of internal and external factors. I could be exercising religiously, but also get injured when I am training for a competition and overdo things. And let's not even talk about andropause or the male menopause, which has slowly been making its presence felt. And yet, I'm learning to embrace my ageing body alongside things I learn from people around me to make sure that I make every day count.

If you have the knowledge and access to resources to allow you to be the best version of yourself, would you actually take concrete steps to seize it? That's the question I want to ask of you before you even begin to read this book. In these pages, you will find interviews and insights from experts from across the globe on everything from sleep to nutrition to training to biohacking and everything in between. I also share with you at length things that I've personally tried or experienced to give you insights from someone who is eternally curious about the workings of the human mind and body, and how to maximize what we've been given to their fullest potential. In the course of writing this book, I've made myself into a human guinea pig in the name of science, and am sharing these with you with as much honesty and sincerity as I can muster in the name of art.

Who am I you may ask? I'm really just an ordinary guy trying to do extraordinary things. If I look at the things I've done in my life, I would say I'm somewhat of an overachiever. I'm not particularly smart or handsome or funny or lucky. But somehow, I always like punching above my weight and if I really want something, I'm willing to put in the work to get it. At some point, I always manage to get it done.

Health and wellness have always been important aspects of my life and something that I've used to define myself as a person. Yes, I identify as a peak performer (physically and emotionally), but I am far from being an 'expert' on the matter. What I've gotten really good at though is taking advice from people through the years that I have either been given or have been inspired by, which I am now sharing in this book.

If you're looking for an inspiring turnaround story like losing a hundred pounds or turning my life around by doing some drastic intervention that changed the course of my life, you have the wrong guy. My life and any modest success I've had is due to doing the right things consistently, generally staying off the bad, and doing things in moderation.

The perspective in this book comes from an eternally curious approach to life, the willingness to try new things, and finding what works at a particular moment in time. The approach is not dogmatic, but rather open and malleable. I am painfully aware that a good number or points explored in this book have a good chance of being irrelevant or even obsolete within even just a span of a few years. But there are also universal truths within these pages that have and will continue to stand the test of time.

Why have I written this book? From a personal standpoint, I wanted to see if I could compile all the things that, as of this book's writing, I could utilize to optimize my performance. Things I've tried to enhance my mind and body, and how to make what I learned not just accessible but also practical and replicable for most people.

I have very big, hairy, audacious goals, and I would like to accomplish them in the one mind and body that I have to work with. Whether it's to build more businesses that can impact more people, my desire to continue competing as a master (another term for an older, really) athlete, or my aspirations to live to a ripe old and healthy age of a hundred years old.

From a health and wellness perspective, I've always been curious about the right things to do that help optimize physical and mental health and well-being. I've had many struggles, injuries, and self-doubt. I've also had to deal with my insecurities and this nagging impostor syndrome. Do I have what it takes to continuously be successful in navigating the different areas of my life? I've persisted though, and in this book, I've documented how and take you through my most honest assessment of the peak performance protocols that I have found and, in most cases, tried.

I am fortunate to have travelled the world and worked with experts from different fields and tried different approaches to attaining physical and mental peak performance. But what good is an amazing journey if you can't share it with other people? It is my hope that through this book, you will be able to join me in this quest and find your own path towards fulfilling your peak performance goals. In these pages I've shared very personal experiences, training regimens, insights, and even medical records and results from my diagnostics for you to see what a comprehensive assessment of health and fitness can look like.

I've fucked things up along the way and maybe if I share some of these things, you can learn a thing or two, so you don't make the same mistakes. But if you do, heck, we're all works in progress anyway.

If you're ready, we'll begin with the first and most important lesson. A good night's sleep.

Disclaimer

This book is an ambitious exploration that spans countries, cultures, and demographics to unravel the practical approach to attaining human peak performance. This book delves into the author's personal journey, as he embarks on a transformative quest to optimize his mind and body.

John's immersion allows him to test the protocols and lessons he uncovers, making him an interesting case study for human peak performance. This book is a fusion of scientific and medical principles, personal experimentation, and cross-cultural sociological insights that guide readers toward the methods to live their lives to their longest and fullest potential.

The exercises, nutritional recommendations, and lifestyle strategies discussed in this book are based on the author's research and experience. Remember that individual health conditions and fitness levels vary, and it is crucial to consult a healthcare professional before attempting any new exercise programme or making significant changes to your diet.

The contents of this book should not be considered a substitute for professional medical advice, diagnosis, or treatment. Always seek the advice of your physician or other qualified health provider with any questions you may have regarding a medical condition. The author and publisher disclaim any liability for any injuries or health issues that may arise from the use of the information provided.

Readers are advised to use their discretion and carefully consider their own health status before implementing any suggestions from this book. There are very real dangers that one may incur health complications or even die as a result of following some of the practices in this book. It is recommended to consult qualified sports and healthcare professionals for personalized advice tailored to individual circumstances.

Health is a personal responsibility, and decisions regarding well-being should be made in consultation with qualified healthcare professionals.

Chapter 1

Sleep

'When I wake up, I am reborn.'

—Mahatma Gandhi

Sleep, bar none, is the single most important component of health of any human being. It is the underrated elixir of youth, the ultimate health hack, the basic building block and foundation of well-being.

Long gone is the belief that sleep is for the weak. The founder of what was once a little startup called Amazon, Jeff Bezos, admits that though he gets up at 5 or 6 a.m., he always makes it a priority to get a full eight hours of sleep. Mark Zuckerberg does the same. Even Elon Musk upped his sleep hours to six from his previously unhealthy sometimes all-nighters.

From an economic perspective, following these billionaires' examples in getting a good night's sleep would definitely be a smart move; research compiled by SleepFoundation.org suggests that, just in the US, insufficient sleep has an economic impact of over $411 billion, with $31.1 billion being linked to insomnia-related workplace errors and accident costs.[1]

In terms of sleep's impact on one's overall physical well-being, The National Council on Aging (NCOA) cites research that states how inadequate sleep puts one at a higher risk for heart-related diseases, and other ailments such as Type 2 diabetes, high blood pressure, obesity, stroke, and even early death. There is also the toll that lack of sleep takes on one's mental health, wherein those with inadequate shuteye being two and a half times more likely to experience frequent mental distress.[2]

Sleep is the first chapter of this book on peak performance because it is, arguably, the most important factor in personal optimization, and one that we all rely on at the most basic level.

I admit my relationship with sleep has been contentious to say the least, and one that can either be totally predictable and routinary, or the opposite extreme. There have been points in my life when sleep came easy, and I would have no problems whatsoever. There have also been stretches when it was elusive and I tried different remedies, with varying levels of success. For something that we should be doing for at least one third of our lives, it is incumbent upon each person to understand how to do this one activity best.

Instead of glorifying muscles and curves and someone's Vo2 Max, we should be envious of someone who gets to sleep at 8.30 p.m. and sleeps more than eight hours a night. Now, that's sexy.

So, what exactly happens to our mind and body during sleep?

First, we need to understand our circadian rhythm, or how we are 'tuned to the daily cycle of night and day', and the physical, mental, and behavioural changes that we experience over a period of twenty-four hours. In simpler terms, one's circadian rhythm is controlled by a 'master clock' in the brain, that tells us when we should sleep and wake up.[3]

That circadian rhythm can be disrupted by a number of things, most commonly by irregular sleep hours (think: night shift workers, travellers with jet lag), and by the blue light in electronic gadgets.

Assuming that your circadian rhythm is in sync, getting a good night's sleep means going through the two kinds of sleep: Non-Rapid Eye Movement (NREM) and Rapid Eye Movement (REM). As you close your eyes, you first enter NREM sleep, which is divided into three or four stages, says world renowned sleep authority Matthew

Walker, PhD, an author, speaker, and professor of Neuroscience and Psychology at the University of California, Berkeley, and founder and director of the Center for Human Sleep Science:[4]

Table 1.1: Stages of sleep

Stages of Sleep According to Matthew Walker	
NREM	Stage 1 - Awake/Light Sleep
	Stage 2 - Light Sleep
	Stage ¾ - Deep Sleep
REM	'Paradoxical Sleep' - Dream Sleep

As you go through each stage, sleep gets deeper, and it is in deep sleep when one's immunity is 'recharged', the cardiovascular system gets an overhaul, and memories are imprinted in the brain. REM sleep is when one's creativity gets a boost, and where one experiences a lot of brainwave activity (this is when we see a lot of eye movement even though the body is completely paralyzed—hence the name, and why it's called paradoxical), as the brain 'stitches' information gathered throughout our waking hours.

We go through these stages of sleep every ninety minutes, and they form one's sleep architecture. However, the ratio of NREM and REM sleep within the ninety-minute cycle varies throughout the night, in such a way that during the first half of our sleep, we get more of the NREM type, while in the second half, we get to experience more REM sleep. Walker emphasizes that it is important to get enough of both, as deprivation of either results in all types of physical and mental dysfunction, which, peak performer or not, is something you would want to avoid.[5]

It is undeniable that there are very grave, even fatal, repercussions of having not enough sleep, or being totally deprived of it. There are daredevils, such as American seventeen-year-old

Randy Gardner, who set the world record in 1963 when he went eleven days and twenty minutes without sleep, but studies have consistently shown that sleep deprivation can put one's mental clarity, memory, immune system, cardiovascular system, metabolism, and mental health at risk.[6]

In the following pages, I have put together a compendium of what has worked for myself and many people, including experts in the field. My goal is for you to be able to carve out from a twenty-four-hour day the ideal number of hours of sleep you need to enable you to perform at your absolute best. If you're ready, let's begin with the first minute.

The Morning Ritual for a Good Night's Sleep

Ironically, getting a good night's sleep starts the moment you wake up.

There are a number of people that I have been following through the years, none more impactful to my sleep and morning daily ritual than neuroscientist Dr Andrew Huberman,[7] known as the podcaster who 'got America to care about science'. Also a Stanford School of Medicine associate professor, Huberman hosts Huberman Lab, one of the top health podcasts in the US. His much-followed morning protocol has spurred numerous videos on YouTube documenting how they 'did the Andrew Huberman morning routine for X days/ weeks and this is what happened'.

When people start writing and vlogging about following something that you do that makes them want to change their life, you know your research and protocol has reached a certain cult status where people have sat up, listened to, and actually done the work.

One of the main things that Huberman discusses in his work is how to set up one's self throughout the day so you can get a good night's sleep at the end of it.[8] I have followed his advice and created this morning ritual for myself, with my own personal assessment and with feedback from other experts.

Routine 1: Wake up early

Ideally, it's wise to start your day early, and that is because of the hormone cortisol. Largely seen as a stress hormone, cortisol is a key driver that pushes you to wake up from sleep—and it is best that this hormone is released early in the day. This is called a 'cortisol pulse', and this will dictate the timing of the release of melatonin, the hormone that will help you fall asleep at night, which usually happens twelve to fourteen hours after the cortisol pulse.

The discipline to wake up at 6 a.m. every morning is due mainly to the fact that I take my nine-year-old son to school. Once your body gets used to waking up early, it's hard to wake up later even if you wanted to, and we all know this. The key is how to keep this regularity even on weekends. For people who spend their Friday and Saturday evenings out late and perhaps consuming inebriating substances, or perhaps sleeping in longer than you would during weekdays, waking up early can pose a bit of a challenge. Keeping a consistent wake up time, however, also enables you to have a consistent wind down and sleep schedule at night.

Routine 2: Hydration and delayed caffeine intake

Hydration: drink a glass of lemon water with salt.

I start my day by drinking a glass of lemon water with a pinch of Himalayan salt. This combination helps my body reach optimal hydration first thing in the morning. The salt provides me with the electrolytes I need to remineralize my body and boost my energy levels. The lemon, on the other hand, not only contains Vitamin C but also helps facilitate the digestion process and cleanses my system. This routine is definitely the easiest to stick to because you can have all these ready to be consumed first thing in the morning upon waking up.

Helene Patounas, a clinical and performance nutritionist who works with Hintsa Performance, an evidence-based coaching company that has in its roster of clients Formula 1 Champions and

Fortune 500 CXOs, says this is also part of her morning routine. In an interesting conversation about nutrition (which we'll dive deeper into in the next chapter), she shares with me how she would have warm lemon water to help with bowel movement and get vital nutrients in, as lemon is also good for cleansing one's liver. She does warn, however, that lemon can have an effect on one's tooth enamel, so one should also be conscious of lemon's effect on your teeth. I find it takes a little bit more work, but you can always swish non-lemon water immediately after you drink the lemon water.

As for Himalayan salt, she says the minerals in it are very helpful in helping the body absorb and utilize water more efficiently—as long as one has no issues with high blood pressure. Of course, I understand that accessibility to this ingredient may vary and Huberman recommends even just a pinch of table salt in one's morning water, also with the caveat that you don't have any problems with your blood pressure.

Tip: Delay caffeine intake ninety to one-twenty minutes upon waking up

Getting in one's morning cup of joe doesn't necessarily need to happen early in the day. In fact, Huberman says you don't have to have caffeine in the morning, especially if you are prone to panic or anxiety attacks.

But for those of you who enjoy caffeine in the form of coffee or tea as you start your day, he recommends waiting at least an hour and a half to two hours upon waking up. The reason for this is linked to cortisol, a hormone naturally released by the body when we wake up—which is why technically, early in the day, you don't need the help of caffeine to perk yourself up. It could also interfere with the release of cortisol and lead you to depend too much on it if you get used to taking your coffee too early in the morning.

Huberman also says that delaying one's caffeine intake by ninety to one-twenty minutes will help you avoid that 'afternoon crash', which typically leads you to drink more caffeine later in the day and sets you up for poor sleep later in the night.

I must admit that it can get really tempting most days to just down that coffee to get the drowsiness out of the way and to get your day started with the jolt of caffeine, but I discovered that delaying it a bit isn't so bad. The in-between can actually be a good time to do the next routine that wakes you up anyway.

Routine 3: Expose yourself to the morning sun.

One of the most common newborn care practices taught to parents is to bring out their baby during sunrise—ideally before 8 a.m.—and for good reason: it's one of the best times to catch the longest wavelength of light, along with sunset. Sun exposure is a biohacking technique, says Eli Abela of Bulletproof Human Potential, that doesn't just boost one's Vitamin D, but has also helped people resolve a number of health issues. 'There are actually stories where people go out to sunrise and sunset for months, and have healed their vision problems, depression, or anything else that they need,' says Abela, a biohacking pioneer and top vitality coach in the Philippines. 'There's just a sense of well-being when you come out into nature at the time where the skies are pink and violet and yellow and just beautiful.'

Waking up to catch the morning sun also sets up a timer of sorts for the time you will fall asleep at night, says Huberman, through the trigger of the release of cortisol in your brain. Getting morning sunlight increases early-day cortisol release (which is the ideal time for elevated cortisol) and getting sunlight in your system early in the day can boost that, which helps improve your immune system and alertness and prepares the body for sleep later that night. That timer to fall asleep, says Huberman, usually kicks in fourteen to sixteen hours later.

I find the best way to do this is by going to my backyard and just basking in the sun's rays most mornings. I try to put a moisturizing sunblock on my face, but make sure as much of my skin as possible is exposed to the sun, at least for five to ten minutes. For those who believe that the sun is bad for you (and it is in excess especially midday when the sun is at its harshest), I fully respect your opinions and beliefs. I am just at a point right now when moderation for me is key in life, a theme that you will find throughout this book as key to my search for the art and science of peak performance. For those living in countries that get minimal sunlight, I share with you an alternative: red light therapy through the redbed. Read more about it in Chapter 7, where I share other techniques you can employ that go beyond traditional health protocols.

Routine 4: Meditate

Practice this to start your day in an emotionally calm state, and to clear your mind, even for just three to five minutes. You can do focused meditation, which involves placing specific attention on your breath, body, or a mental visualization. You can also do mindfulness meditation; in which case you allow your thoughts to come and go without attachment.

Though I don't do this consciously, mindfulness meditation seems to be my automatic state of mind most mornings as I stare out into our pool and garden. Being close to nature, water in particular, is immensely helpful in calming the mind. I've naturally gravitated towards this practice and just let my mind wander without any clear direction or agenda. I have in the past tried to be a bit more structured by actually doing some form of meditation exercise but found that I am better off just having a blank mind and allowing myself to receive thoughts and give time for the silence and serenity of the morning.

Routine 5: Move

Movement and exercise are hallmarks to many peak performers' morning routine. This can range anywhere from a short stroll to stretching exercises to a full-blown workout, depending on your preference. Huberman, for example, likes to do 'forward ambulation', or simply put, taking a walk outside.[9] Any forward ambulation, he says, whether that's walking or biking or running, gives us an optic flow, or a 'visual streaming' that has a positive effect on our amygdala—helping reduce our stress and anxiety. He also says that early morning exercise, or exercise done within one to three hours after waking, also sets one up for mental alertness throughout the day, because of the release of neurochemicals triggered by physical activity.[10]

I am cognizant of the fact, however, that some people—myself included—prefer to work out or exercise later in the day, and this is really a matter of personal preference and circumstance. Having some form of movement though, no matter how little early in the morning, can do wonders for your ability to face the day on a positive note.

Other Protocols

There are other protocols that Huberman does such as deep work, journalling, and cold exposure, that are really dependent on your personal life circumstances which you can try if it makes sense and works for you. There have been many who tried Huberman's morning routine, with varying levels of success and failure. At the end of the day do take from it what you need without feeling pressured to take it as bible truth as we are all made different.

Evening Ritual: Protecting Your Sleep

Your evening ritual, suggests Helene Patounas, should focus on doing things pre-bedtime that would 'protect' your sleep, so you get the right quality and amount of shuteye that the body needs to recharge. For Chien Han How, a medical entrepreneur who founded the Sleepwake Centre in Singapore—and a guest/subject matter expert featured in my podcast and previous book *Methods to Greatness*—the same is true. He recommends getting into a relaxed state before going to sleep, and working on your 'sleep hygiene', which essentially is about timing one's sleep schedule so that your body naturally cues you on when it is time to go to bed and when it is time to wake up.

Some of the things you can do are to:

- **Time your last meal and fluid intake**.
  Dr Andrew Huberman recommends that you don't eat too close to bedtime, but to not go to sleep hungry, either. Leading performance coach and best-selling author Brendon Burchard's 3-2-1 Rule is something that's good to follow, too: No food three hours before sleep, no water two hours before sleep, and no devices one hour before sleep.[11]

  I don't starve myself for dinner, and since I became more conscious of not eating anything after that, no eating three hours before sleep is very doable for me. What I find particularly annoying is the fact that prior to me discovering this sleep hack, I would get up two, sometimes three, times a night because I have to pee. Since I started being more conscious of timing my last fluid intake, this has been drastically reduced to once a night, sometimes not even.

  I am also well aware of the fact that my sleep is not as restful when I have a late meal. For a 10 p.m. sleep target, our family always makes it a point to eat before 7 p.m., which ensures that our bodies have adequate time to wind down. Midnight snacks are a definite no-no.

- **Limit your caffeine eight to ten hours before your bedtime.**
  Matthew Walker says that ten hours would be the ideal window, but if you want to push it, eight is the limit. That's because of caffeine's effect on your adenosine—a byproduct of cellular metabolism, which you accumulate throughout the day—and how it is responsible for making you sleepy at the end of that day. Caffeine is an adenosine receptor blocker, and according to Walker, when the brain can't detect the correct level of adenosine in your system, it starts to think that you haven't been awake for, say, twelve hours, and

therefore won't need to sleep just yet. Taking coffee later in the day, or at night, will therefore affect the duration of your sleep; and even if you are able to still sleep after a shot of espresso at 8 p.m., you will have poor sleep quality, says Walker, as you won't be able to achieve that much-needed deep sleep.

I know this only too well from experience, and make sure not to have anything caffeinated after lunch. The times that I do, I end up regretting it as I don't have that automatic drowsy feeling close to bedtime.

- **Step into a sauna.**
  If you have access to one nearby or have one at home, a twenty-minute sauna session in the evening, capped off with a quick cold shower will bring your body temperature down and set you up for sleep. No sauna? No problem. A hot shower or bath will also do the trick.

  Our sauna at home is one of the best health investments we've ever made. It will pay for itself with the number of extra hours of sleep you will get at night because it will knock you out and give you a sweet slumber, especially if you do it in the evening. My routine consists of at least a thrice a week sauna session late in the day, usually after a workout. It's amazing how sleepy I actually get on the days that I do a sauna session. Even if I do the session earlier in the day, the sauna gives me the same feeling of wanting to drift off into a nice slumber by bedtime.

- **Set up your environment for sleep.**
  - Get cool. The temperature of your room can affect how well you sleep. Cooling down the room also lowers your body temperature, which is what you need to be able to fall asleep easily.

○ Turn off or remove your device/s. As previously mentioned, screen time should be avoided at least an hour before you settle in to sleep, because of exposure to blue light, or, if you must use it, put on blue-light blocking glasses. That's because this kind of light can stimulate alertness in our brain, which therefore disrupts our circadian rhythm by essentially making us think that it is still daytime.[12] Moreover, these devices create electromagnetic fields (EMF), and research has shown the continued exposure to EMF contributes to poorer sleep quality, as well as depression and anxiety. I personally put my phone in our walk-in closet just across our room, as far away from our bed as possible.

○ Avoid bright light and use dimmer lighting in the evenings, as doing so can promote the production of melatonin and improve sleep quality. In the same vein, you can also minimize all other sources of light by using blackout window shades or even a sleep mask.

Apart from taking these steps, other factors that can help you fall and stay asleep easier:

- **Sex**
  According to Walker, there is data to support that sex where orgasm occurs, as well as masturbation, has sleep benefits, as related to the hormone oxytocin, which gets you ready for rest. He also points out that as with other activities, the reverse is the same—better sleep improves sexual behaviour, in the same way that a good diet and adequate exercise promotes better sleep.

  Some fun facts: An extra hour of sleep increases libido by 14 per cent, while quality sleep optimizes sex hormones.

Masturbation can increase sleep quality by 47 per cent and help you fall asleep faster. I think we all know this, people. At least, now, you understand the science.

- **Avoid alcohol**

  While alcohol is a depressant that can sedate you enough to help you fall asleep quickly, taking it close to bedtime will give you poor quality sleep, and affect your wakefulness the following day. If you must drink in the evening, make sure that you stop at least four hours before bedtime, so your body has time to metabolize the alcohol in your system.[13]

- **Meditation**

  Huberman classifies meditation as a nonsleep deep rest (NSDR) practice, 'guide your brain and body into a state of deep relaxation without falling asleep completely.' Aside from meditation, there's also yoga nidra or yogic sleep, as well as hypnosis and breathwork. There are also many apps that you can use for meditation and sleep aid such as Headspace and Calm, and you just have to choose what works best for you.

The Power of Napping

Who doesn't love a midday nap? My personal rule of thumb is that if I feel sleepy midday, I know my body is telling me something that I should listen to, and just go with it. Most times, I feel much better after.

Matthew Walker says that physiologically, humans typically experience a dip in energy and alertness mid-afternoon, between 1–4 p.m. He says that while many in first-world nation practice 'monophasic' sleep, or one long sleep stretch at night, a closer look at this 'preprogrammed' behaviour of midday sleepiness suggests that what we need is 'biphasic' sleep, or sleep that is divided into two parts, with one occurring for a short period (around twenty minutes, to avoid going into deep sleep during daytime),[14] and a longer period at night.[15] He also highlights that around the world, many nations have a siesta culture, and that the benefits of naps are undeniable: aside from reducing daytime sleepiness, it helps one focus, boosts learning and performance, and improves alertness.[16]

It's no wonder 'power nap' became a term we use to describe the refreshed feeling we get after a quick snooze. An ideal duration for a nap is between ten to thirty minutes; any longer than that and you will experience sleep inertia, or that feeling of grogginess and fatigue that you likely wanted to get rid of in the first place by napping.[17]

However, Walker also calls taking a midday nap a 'double-edged sword', as it can potentially have a negative effect on your nighttime sleep. Remember adenosine? If you are the type of person who can't fall asleep easily at night, Walker recommends that you avoid daytime napping, so you can have a healthy buildup of adenosine in your system, that will pressure your body to fall asleep when you need to at the end of the day.

Minus that factor, naps come highly recommended by Walker and other sleep experts. Try to squeeze one in before 2 p.m., so you're still doing it early enough and not taking anything away from your longer sleep in the evening.

Sleep Banking

If nap time seems hardwired in our biology, think of sleep banking as more of a strategy, one that has been adopted by peak performers across the world, including the military.[18] Also called 'sleep extension', banking entails that you anticipate instances when you expect to be sleep-deprived, and therefore add a couple more hours of sleep to the nights leading up to those instances. Studies show that benefits of sleep banking include a more sustained attention span and reduced sleep pressure, and, in moments of sleep deprivation, helps in one's psychomotor performance.[19]

Even best-selling author Tim Ferris has been advised by performance coach Andy Galpin, in his podcast interview on *The Tim Ferris Show*,[20] on the advantages of sleep banking. He mentions the need for sleep banking when going into high-intensity training or fight camps (hence this strategy's usefulness to the military), but also highlights its usefulness outside of the context of sleep deprivation, and 'maximizing' sleep so you can get ahead of the high-performance tasks expected of you. He says studies have shown that adding anywhere from forty-five minutes a night for three days or sleeping for ten hours for five to seven weeks ahead has improved performance in athletes such as rugby players, high-endurance cyclists, and division one basketball players.

Moreover, Galpin cites a study led by Cheri D. Mah, a clinical and translational research fellow at the University of California San Francisco (UCSF) Human Performance Center and UCSF School of Medicine, which states that athletes who are already getting in the right amount of sleep, benefit greatly from sleep extension that is done on top of their healthy, habitual nightly sleep. Positive effects observed from those who participated in the study include 'improvements in shooting percentage, sprint times, reaction time, mood, fatigue, and vigour.'[21]

Monitoring Sleep Health and the Use of Wearables

In the past, sleep health has been measured only in labs, requiring one to spend the night hooked up to machines while being recorded on video. This also usually happens when one has a sleep issue that needs resolving, or a disorder that needs to be understood better to find the right treatment.

Wearable medical devices, i.e. sleep trackers, changed the game and gave us access to our own personal 'sleep labs' at home. Now, we are able to get real-time insights on our sleeping patterns, heart rate, and breathing patterns, and this information can help us better understand what our body needs.

On a larger scale, the data that wearables have been able to gather also reveal interesting insights about people's current general health habits, which, aside from sleep, include exercise and overall lifestyle. According to Janne Kallio, head of partner products at Suunto—Finnish manufacturer of performance watches—some of these insights show how, for example, many people generally have poor sleep on New Year's Eve (for obvious reasons). The relevance of this data, he told me during my interview with him in Helsinki, is its impact on the company's scientific research to understand how to train more efficiently and identify correlations between lifestyle factors and health.

The WHOOP strap and Oura Ring are two commonly used fitness trackers that record real-time data and provide insights for those who want to track the quality of their sleep and overall wellness. The Oura ring is something I've personally tried only recently; as of this book's writing I've been able to get close to a years' worth of information on my health. My curiosity around wearables started when I was having a particularly hard time getting enough sleep and would wake up at three or four in the morning. It started during the pandemic when existential questions started rearing their ugly heads and the restless 'monkey mind' started taking over.

I find that the ring form factor makes sense for a sleep tracker. Some of the data that the Oura ring shows me is:[22]

- **Sleep data**
  Your total time asleep and how much time in each stage (awake, REM, light, deep).

- **Resting heart rate**
  The number of times your heart beats in a minute when you are at rest.
- **Heart Rate Variability (HRV)**
  Your heart's adaptability to different situations and stress levels.
- **Resilience**
  Your ability to withstand physiological stress, and also recover from it.
- **Readiness**
  A holistic picture of your overall health based on the aforementioned data.

It's been fascinating to track my sleep and other health patterns from just wearing a ring and finding a wealth of insights on my mobile phone. It's a great way to keep track of your sleep and help you prepare for and plan your day as well. It has helped me make decisions such as not training heavily (if at all) on a day when I didn't get enough sleep the previous night, taking a nap to increase my sleep score, and meditating in the middle of the day to lower my daytime stress levels.

Janne emphasized in our conversation, however, that while wearables give us great data, there is still the challenge of missing contextual information about users, such as the effect of their diet and other factors, which can impact the interpretation of the data.

Sleep Requirements Based on Age

Most sleep experts recommend a full eight hours of sleep for the average adult, but, as most of us know, the sleep we require changes throughout life.[23] Here's a quick snapshot:

Table 1.2: Different age groups and the hours of sleep they require
on a regular basis [24]

Age	Number of sleep hours per 24 hours, on a regular basis
4–12 months	12–16 hours, including naps
1–2 years old	11–14 hours, including naps
3–5 years old	10–13 hours, including naps
6–12 years old	9–12 hours
13–18 years old	8–10 hours
18–60 years old	At least 7 hours

Sleep Hacking: Adjusting Your Sleep Time

Before we close this chapter, I'd like to also share a useful tip for those who find themselves needing to adjust their sleep time, either because they're travelling across multiple time zones often, or have to keep irregular hours for other reasons—work, caring for kids or other loved ones. Again, taking wisdom from Huberman, take note of these two words: **temperature minimum**. It refers to when your body is at its lowest temperature in the twenty-four-hour cycle, which typically occurs two hours before you normally wake up in the morning. Using that as your reference point, you can help your body adjust to a changing sleep schedule or perform a 'phase shift to your circadian clock'.

Phase advance

If you want to shift your circadian rhythm earlier, you should expose yourself to bright light shortly after your new wake up time, ideally within thirty minutes of the temperature minimum. This early morning light exposure helps signal to your body that it's time to wake up and initiates the internal processes that synchronize with the new wake-up time. Additionally, you should avoid bright light exposure in the evening, especially close to bedtime, as it can delay the release of melatonin, the hormone that regulates sleep. Additionally, consider increasing the ambient temperature in your environment, such as by turning up the thermostat or taking a warm shower. Higher temperatures can complement the wake-up signals from light exposure, further encouraging your body to transition into an alert state.

Phase delay

Conversely, if you aim to shift your circadian rhythm later, you should minimize exposure to bright light in the morning. This lack of morning light exposure signals to your body that it's not yet time to wake up, thus delaying the onset of the wake-up phase. In the evening, you can expose yourself to bright light, especially in the hours leading up to bedtime, as this can help suppress melatonin release and promote wakefulness. Consider maintaining a cool ambient temperature in your environment up to your new wake up time and delaying cooling your environment during the night to help facilitate a delay in the circadian rhythm. Cooler temperatures can complement the lack of morning light exposure, reinforcing the signals for extended sleep.

If you are travelling, first determine which direction you are going—when travelling eastward, you 'phase advance'. This means that you're moving across time zones where the local time is ahead of your original time zone. As a result, you need to adjust your circadian rhythm to align with the new time zone, essentially advancing your sleep-wake cycle earlier. The reverse is true when travelling westward.

The same concept applies when shifting to a new work schedule, but ideally, if you're doing swing shifts, make sure you stick to a schedule for at least two weeks before changing, so as not to make things worse for your sleep health.

We can also learn a thing or two on sleep optimization from the experts who optimize sleep for F1 racers.

Hintsa Performance is an evidence-based coaching company based in Finland that has in its roster of clients Formula 1 Champions and Fortune 500 CXOs from around the world. In an interview in Helsinki with Pekka Pohjakallio, director and executive mentor at Hintsa Performance, I learned that evening races such as the Singapore Grand Prix pose unique challenges to drivers who are more accustomed to racing during the day. Instead of trying to adapt to the local time zone, Pekka says coaches simply simulate conditions similar to those in the drivers' home countries. They do this by taking drivers to brightly lit areas in the evening when they get to Singapore, such as malls, to mimic daylight exposure, while blackout curtains ensure a conducive sleep environment during the day.

By carefully managing exposure to light and other factors that influence the body's circadian rhythm, coaches help drivers maintain peak performance levels despite the time difference.

My Personal Challenges

As I mentioned, my relationship with sleep has been contentious through the years, and I believe it will remain so, as long as I am on this unpredictable journey called life.

I've established my morning and bedtime routine as much as I can. The Oura rings that my wife Monica and I gave to each other as Christmas gifts have allowed us to better track our sleep. After checking my weight, I check my sleep—how long or little I've slept and how ready my body is to face the day ahead. One has to be mindful though of just how fanatical you can tend to be when you monitor your sleep. Monica tells me that she sometimes feels anxious when the Oura ring gives her a low sleep or resilience score, which perhaps causes her to be more stressed, thus affecting her numbers further.

This reminds me of what another Hintsa performance coach, Malaysia-based Matti Kontsas shared with me, that getting a good night's sleep goes beyond setting a perfect routine. It's not a performance, but a time to relax. 'We can build this perfect performance routine in a sense, and, in theory, it can be good for your sleep, but it can be another source of stress because it's another thing that [you] have to do,' he explains.

Still, I've made some inroads in improving my sleep quality with the things I've learned. In the evenings, I've tried to protect my sleep by not eating anything after dinner. We've also installed smart lighting in our bedroom that allows us to automatically dim the lights at a certain time to help prepare us for sleep. Additionally, I make sure to keep our room as dark as possible and even use an eye mask for added measure.

We still have a nine-year-old boy who stays with us in our room and refuses to share the 'boy's room' with our other twenty-year-old son. So, after reading to him, he stays a few more minutes on our bed before he transfers to his mattress on the floor. We've been saying for years that this year would be the last since this arrangement really hampers our sleep, but it is what it is. We're just trying to enjoy the last year(s) that he still wants to be close and snuggle with his parents.

While we do our best to maintain good sleep hygiene, life is unpredictable and ensuring a good night's sleep every night for the rest of your life is an unreasonable expectation. However, we can take into account our compromised state when lacking sleep, and prepare to encounter the day accordingly. Just last year, I sustained a hamstring injury last that I know was definitely due in part to not getting enough sleep the previous night. I had to be in the CNN Philippines studios very early to promote my last book, and I probably only got around four hours of sleep. The afternoon of that day, despite how I felt, I went ahead and did my sprints training and subsequently strained my hamstrings, which necessitated two weeks of rehab.

These days, I'm a lot more conscious and cautious when it comes to protecting my sleep, as it directly affects how much load I can put on my body. From my Oura numbers, I've come to realize how much of an impact factors such as my last meal in the evening, alcohol, and travelling can have on my sleep. I've also done some experiments and fine tuning on what I can do to optimize it. The best sleep hacks that work for me? Exercise, sauna, some 'Netflix and chill' with the wifey, and reading a book to our son.

Your to-do list to achieve peak sleep:

- **Set your sleep routine and get things in order by doing a room makeover.**
  Set up thick or blackout curtains, install soft lights, and make sure your room is nice and cold.
- **Find a place outside the bedroom where you can place your phone.**
  It should be well away from your reach, but still within earshot in case of emergencies.
- **Instead of grabbing a cup of coffee after lunch, take a nap.**
  If your schedule and circumstances permit it, squeeze in a power nap (ten–thirty minutes) in the middle of the day when you are feeling drowsy instead of downing coffee.
- **Explore sleep tracking options that are most accessible for you.**
  Use this to get a better understanding of your sleep patterns, and to improve your sleep quality.

Chapter 2

Nutrition and Supplementation

Food and its consumption by the human species has been changing for thousands of years. From being hunters and gatherers, humans changed how they nourished themselves with the Agricultural Revolution, which took place around 10,000 years ago. From there, we built and grew and birthed modern society as we know it. About 100 years ago, the Industrial Revolution, or the Second Agricultural Revolution, as Yuval Noah Harari calls it in his book *Sapiens: A Brief History of Humankind*,[25] again changed how we approached food production.

In the next 100 years, what do you suppose our food would look like and what would our relationship with it be?

Dr Lauri Reuter, a specialist in cell biology, genetic engineering, and protein production, and an alumnus of the Singularity University Global Solutions Program 2017, looks at it from a food production security perspective. I listened to his eye-opening insights when I attended Singularity University in Silicon Valley in 2019. I learned that with climate change, and at the rate that the world is consuming food, we need to rethink the way we eat,[26] and what we eat, starting with the idea that we can possibly do away with animal-based products. Beyond plant-based alternatives, think of using artificial intelligence to create food from scratch, based on our specific needs collected by the wearable devices that contain all our health information. This would give us freedom from choice, as

Dr Reuter puts it, since so far, having multiple food choices has led us towards the lifestyle diseases we experience today.

But whether we think about the past, present, or future, what we eat plays a role on how we perform physically and mentally every day, more so if you are striving to achieve peak performance. In this chapter, we'll dive into our relationship with food—and how we can make the best choices in order to become the best version of ourselves.

Popular Diet Trends

When it comes to the way we eat, we all know how greatly the agricultural revolution changed the way the human race lived— from being constantly on the move to hunt or gather our food, we learned to grow them, enabling civilizations to flourish and establish roots. Since then, our food consumption has become influenced by more complicated factors: our income level, urbanization, trade liberalization, global food corporations (and their food processing systems), food retailing (think large supermarket chains), food marketing, and, of course, consumer attitudes and behaviour.[27]

Part of these consumer attitudes and behaviour is our gravitation towards diets that promote healthy eating habits or, for those seeking it, weight loss.

From counting calories, juicing, fasting intermittently, going vegan, and even reviving our cavemen ancestors' eating habits, it's hard to ignore the diet trends that have prevailed over the decades, with some gaining many high-profile ambassadors and believers. We can't deny the way these diet trends have influenced how we nourish ourselves, and, ultimately, our relationship with food. Here are a few that have become quite popular around the world, to help give perspective to where we are now.

Table 2.1: The efficacy of different diets

Diet	How it works	Effects
Grapefruit aka Hollywood diet	Low-calorie diet that involves eating grapefruit during mealtimes, because of the belief that it has fat-burning properties.	Grapefruit can make you feel full and well-hydrated despite having a limited number of calories, yes, but it doesn't increase one's fat metabolism.[28] It is classified by the Academy of Nutrition and Dietetics as a 'monotonous' diet that could make you miss out on necessary nutrients.[29]
Master Cleanse, introduced by alternative health advocate Stanley Burroughs	Ten to forty-five day detox programme where one takes only lemon juice mixed with maple syrup, water, and cayenne pepper.	Studies have shown that while this diet helps one to lose weight, it's only in the short-term.[30] Like other detox diets, it also robs you of enriching yourself with the right amount of daily calories and nutrients.
Atkins and South Beach Diet	This diet focuses on carbohydrate restriction.	Data on the efficacy of both diets in terms of long-term weight loss isn't strong as they still produce more short-term results.

Palaeolithic diet aka Paleo	Eat how the cavemen ate: fresh food such as vegetables, fruits, seeds, and nuts, as well as lean meat and fish. No modern, processed products, whole grains, cereals, dairy, white potatoes, legumes, alcohol, coffee, salt, and refined grains, sugars, and vegetable oils.	Jury's still out on the long-term benefits, and how the exclusion of certain food affects one's nutrient requirements.[31]
Ketogenic diet aka Keto	Restricts one's carbohydrate intake, and allows for a more fat-rich diet, which deprives the body of glucose (from carbs) and triggers the production of ketones, and, subsequently, initiates ketosis to aid in weight loss.[32]	Short-term results have been seen, but long-term effects, as well safety issues—consuming a high-fat diet also has its repercussions—are yet to be determined.
Plant-Based diets (vegan and vegetarian)	A vegan diet excludes all animal-based products while a vegetarian diet allows for some, such as dairy, eggs, fish, and seafood.	Recent studies support plant-based diets as effective for weight loss but must be focused on consuming the right kinds of food—whole foods—versus unhealthy alternatives, such as veggie burgers and sweetened snacks/drinks.[33]

To Be Plant-Based or Not to Be?

The World Health Organization has a library of evidence on the importance of eating your fruits and vegetables every day[34], and recommends that we consume over 400 grams per day to improve our overall health and reduce the risk of noncommunicable diseases. The vitamins and minerals found in this food group, plus dietary fibre, should be enough to convince anyone to get in their daily dose—and there are some, in fact, who have chosen to adapt a diet exclusive to fruits and vegetables, and not just for weight loss.

Bobby Macasaet, chair of the board of directors of Maxicare Health Corporation in the Philippines, is one who has decided to eat plant-based food since 2017—initially to address certain health issues. Bobby was diagnosed with sleep apnoea, which led to a diagnosis of Level 2 prostate cancer. His first step was to immediately eliminate all animal products, including dairy and eggs from his diet. Aside from being cancer-free to this day, by combining cancer treatment with plant-based foods, Bobby tells me has been able to maintain his ideal weight and experience better energy levels allowing him to exercise more and also get better sleep.

'I'm really pleased that I made that decision. It has basically simplified my way of eating. It's not very complicated anymore, and even when I enjoy the company of friends who are not plant-based, I always tell them don't worry, I'll find something on the menu,' he says.

I guess one could say that it was easier for Bobby to adopt a plant-based diet—after all, he has been in the healthcare industry since childhood, as Maxicare was founded by his father, Dr Roberto Macasaet Sr., and would therefore have the right access in terms of nutrition information and food options. But Bobby points out that when he first made the switch seven years ago, there weren't as many vegan choices as we have today; what really motivated him was the desire to take better care of his health.

He shares his tips with me to getting started on a plant-based diet:

- Take baby steps. Try going vegan once a week, for example, by following a 'meatless Mondays' regime.
- Scour your local markets for homegrown produce. There are endless options available. Bobby recommends looking for cruciferous and green leafy vegetables. For snacks, go for beans, seeds, and nuts.
- Do your research. Read up and find a community, because there are others out there who can provide the support you need when adopting a plant-based diet.

Helene has also shared with me that she is an 'advocate of vegetables', because of their anti-ageing properties.[35] 'Vegetables provide carbohydrates, but in very low levels, and they are full of hydrating vitamins and minerals, and of phytonutrients. We now know that every colour represents a new antioxidant or phytonutrient that can have incredible effects even at an epigenetic level; they can do things like switch on and switch off cancer genes,' Helene says. 'Vegetables contain fibre, which is wonderful for gut health as well, and we know now that gut health is central to the overall health of our body.'

And in terms of options, more companies providing meat alternatives are getting the right kind of support, which can only mean more choices for those planning to go vegetarian or vegan. In my previous book and podcast *Methods to Greatness*, I introduced Good Startup and its managing partner Gautam Godhwani, an entrepreneur and investor with over twenty-five years of experience in the technology industry. Good Startup invests in innovations across meat, seafood, dairy, and eggs, as well as materials that come from animals, like wool and silk. He said that by 2025, Asia would be the largest market in the world for alternative proteins, and it is Good Startup's mission to remove animals from the food system through the use of technology.

Gautam believes that going plant-based isn't just healthy for the body, but for the sustainability of the environment. 'The effort here is to really provide consumer choice to give more options to all of us so that we can eat healthier, we can eat in a way that's better for the planet,' he tells me during our interview. 'We can just live our lives in a way that we feel better about.'

Watching the Netflix documentary *Living to 100: Secrets of the Blue Zones* piqued my interest and brought me all the way to Loma Linda in California, known as one of the last remaining Blue Zones in the world. The majority of the population in Loma Linda are seventh-day adventists, who espouse a plant-based diet that's rich in whole foods and excludes most animal products, alcohol, and caffeinated beverages.

An exploration of the Loma Linda Market and a conversation with one of the staff revealed the absence of meat products throughout the entire market. Even the mini cafeteria section serves completely vegan food. Somehow, it felt strange that there was absolutely not a single meat product in this huge grocery market. What they had, however, was an abundance of whole plant foods such as legumes, fruits, vegetables, nuts, and grains. The selection was the widest I have ever seen, and the food in the cafeteria, which I had for lunch, was so good that I didn't even mind that there was absolutely no meat.

If given a wider range of options, would you ever consider going plant-based or weaning yourself away from meat consumption?

Going with Your Gut

To understand exactly what our body needs in terms of nutrition to function at an optimum level, we need to understand where we can get our macro and micronutrients and how they serve us in terms of our goals for endurance and energy, and strength and power. Macronutrients are the nutrients we need to take in large amounts every day to give us the energy we need to perform all our tasks; micronutrients are the vitamins and minerals that we need in small amounts, but have a large impact on our body should we experience a deficit of any one. The following table gives us a good overview of what we need on a daily basis:[36,37,38]

Table 2.2: Nourishment required by our body and where to get it from

Type		Function	Best sources
Macronutrients	Carbohydrates	The brain's primary energy source, which also gets broken down into the glucose needed by the body's cells.	Whole grains (e.g. quinoa, brown rice, oats); starchy vegetables such as sweet potato, corn; bananas, apples, mangoes.
	Protein	Composed of amino acids, which are responsible for the growth, development, repair, and maintenance of body tissue; protects the body's muscles and bones, too.	Lean meat, fish and seafood, beans, lentils, tofu, eggs.
	Fat (polyunsaturated fatty acids: alpha-linolenic and linoleic acid)	Energy storage, hormone production, cell growth, and vitamin absorption.	Fatty fish (e.g. salmon), avocados, canola and olive oils, as well as flax oil, safflower oil, sunflower oil, and corn oil.
	Fibre	Gastrointestinal benefits, reduction of chronic disease risk.	Whole grains, fruits, vegetables.

Micronutrients	Vitamin A	Eye health	Eggs, fish, vegetables, liver of some animal species.

	B Vitamins
	  – Thiamine (B1)
	  – Riboflavin (B2)
	  – Niacin (B3)
	  – Pyridoxine (B6)
	  – Biotin (B8)
	  – Folic Acid (B9)
	  – B12
		Metabolic processes that allow the use of carbohydrates, lipids, and proteins to obtain energy; organ and organ system development, especially the nervous system.	Whole grains, green leafy vegetables, oilseeds, dried fruit, legumes.

	Vitamin C (ascorbic acid)	Antioxidant, protects cells from free radical damage; aids in healing through the biosynthesis of collagen; improves iron absorption from plant-based food.	Fruits (particularly citrus) and vegetables.
	Vitamin K	Coagulation or blood clotting	Green leafy vegetables—spinach, lettuce, broccoli.
	Vitamin D	Calcium absorption and bone tissue synthesis	Sun exposure, cod liver oil, fish, pork liver, eggs, butter.
	Calcium	Development of bone mass	Milk, cheese, yogurt, vegetables.

Phosphorus	Component of bones, teeth, DNA, RNA	Cereals, wholemeal flours, eggs, legumes, fish, milk, cheese, meat.
Iodine	Thyroid hormones synthesis	Iodized salt, cod, tuna, shrimp, seaweed, dairy, eggs.
Iron	Synthesis of haemoglobin in the bone marrow	Meat, fish, cereals, eggs.
Zinc	For growth, immune, and gastrointestinal systems	Meat, fish, seafood—especially oysters.

On top of getting your daily dose of macronutrients and micronutrients, the best nutrition goal one can aim for is to have a healthy gut environment, or microbiome—the ecosystem of good bacteria living in one's intestines. According to the Institute of Functional Medicine (IFM), the health of our gut bacteria affects our whole body, as they help our systems perform many functions, including digestion, balance one's mood, reduce anxiety, and protect against infections.[39]

In my interview with nutrition expert Dr Xiaoran Liu, a professor at Rush University in Chicago, Illinois, she says that one's gut microbiome is influenced by two factors: genes and one's environment, which includes diet, the diversity of microorganisms (which comes from a healthy diet), chemical exposure, and motility, or bowel movement. Taking care of your gut microbiome entails that you maintain a diverse and healthy diet, incorporate prebiotics and probiotics into that diet, manage your use of antibiotics, reduce stress, and exercise regularly. The IFM also lists these tips:

- Eat a wide variety of fibre-rich plant foods, including legumes, nuts, seeds, herbs, whole grains, fruits, and especially vegetables.
- Limit or avoid red meat, processed foods, and foods high in added sugar and artificial sweeteners.
- Stay hydrated. Drink plenty of plain water and other non-caffeinated, unsweetened beverages.
- Limit or avoid any foods to which you are sensitive, intolerant, or allergic.

An unbalanced or unhealthy gut microbiome is usually suffering from dysbiosis[40], which can lead to other conditions such as infections, small intestinal bacterial overgrowth, inflammatory bowel disease, and even atherosclerosis, or the hardening of one's arteries. Aside from poor eating habits, your gut health can also be affected by stress, trauma, surgery, and illness.

While the study of the gut microbiome, according to Dr Liu, is still in its infancy, she notes that one food category stands out when it comes to maintaining a healthy gut: fibre.

'Fibre is really the frontrunner [in a healthy gut microbiome],' Dr Liu tells me. 'And it's whole foods that have high fibre content.'

Fasting: No Hard and Fast Rule

Intermittent fasting, or IF, is one kind of fasting protocol that many people have adopted, especially when it comes to achieving weight loss and achieving metabolic health and longevity. This kind of diet has been called other names as well, such as After 6, wherein one does not eat anything after 6 p.m., and its extreme version OMAD, or the one-meal-a-day diet.

Advocates of fasting would definitely know of Dr Peter Attia, whose extreme fasting regimens—such as going on a seven-day water-only fast once every quarter and a three-day water-only fast once a month—have contributed to the popularity of fasting.

(Attia actually calls IF a misnomer; the term he uses is daily time-restricted feeding, or TR, which is one of three 'levers' in his nutritional framework, the other two being caloric restriction (CR) and dietary restriction (DR). CR refers to how much you eat; DR, what you eat or don't eat; and TR, when you do or don't eat.)

Philip Ruppert, a postdoctoral researcher at the Center for Functional Genomic Studies and Metabolism, Department of Biochemistry and Molecular Biology at the University of Southern Denmark, has broken down the phases of fasting as such: [41]

- **Phase 1**: Food is digested, and the nutrients absorbed and stored in the body.
- **Phase 2**: With the nutrients absorbed into the intestines, the liver gets to work by tapping into its glycogen stores to maintain blood sugar. At the same time, body fat begins releasing fatty acids to fuel the body's energy needs.

- **Phase 3**: The liver's glycogen stores are depleted. The liver starts producing ketones from body fat to fuel the body.

- **Phase 4**: Ketone production is in full swing in the liver, providing the body and the brain with energy. At this point, the body gets almost all its energy from body fat. This phase can last for several weeks.

- **Final phase**: There is no more body fat left. Proteins in the muscle mass are the last resort for obtaining energy to prevent death.

The benefits of fasting, says Ruppert—who authored a review article with Wageningen University and professor Sander Kerseten on the 'Mechanisms of Hepatic Fatty Acid Oxidation and Ketogenesis During Fasting'[42]—include: better energy, sleep, and syncing of one's natural circadian rhythm; more efficient metabolism; improved blood pressure; lower resting heart rate; increased insulin sensitivity; stable blood sugar levels and glowing skin.

He says fasting also helps one be more attuned to what one's body needs, since along the way, you get to learn how your body reacts to your eating and fasting habits.

However, in terms of weight loss, Ruppert says IF doesn't really give you significant results. Attia has also shifted his views on the importance of regular fasting.[43] He no longer does the same level of fasting as he previously did after experiencing loss of muscle mass, which he says isn't worth the trade-off. Over the course of three years, Attia says he lost around ten lbs of muscle mass. He also says that fasting's positive effect on one's health is still difficult to measure on a cellular level.

I admit fasting was not something I personally was into, and only recently started experimenting to see how my body responds to it. I began easy enough with time-restricted feeding, not eating within a twelve-hour period. This is manageable since the goal is just to not eat anything after dinner. So, assuming my last meal is eaten by 7 p.m., a 7 a.m. breakfast does not seem too much of a stretch since I do it anyway. I've learned to just not have any kind of 'midnight snack' or nibble when I'm winding down for bed.

There was a time when hunger pangs would set in and I would have that little snack, which I totally gave up after everything I've been reading and hearing about the benefits of time-restricted eating.

The next step for me was to try and go for about seventeen hours without eating, which means that I would skip breakfast and have lunch as my first meal of the day. I learned to not be so dependent on breakfast, which traditionally has been recommended as the 'biggest meal of the day'.

I've found that since I started fasting, there would be times when I would have breakfast, and it would actually make me feel a bit lethargic as the morning drew on. It would be normal for me to restrict my feeding hours to a heavy lunch, perhaps an afternoon snack prior to a workout capped off by an early dinner. I admit I am quite new to this, but it seems to suit me well.

I've only done a twenty-four-hour fast once. Although I found it to be doable, I don't have the confidence or reason to start doing it on a regular basis yet, since I feel that I need my nutrients whenever I train or exercise, which are usually most days. My goal has always been to be healthier and maintain and not lose weight, especially since I am getting older and would like to retain, if not increase, my muscle mass as I hit my advanced years.

I find that it's easier to fast if you're doing it with someone. My wife was actually the first one who started doing it years ago, and I only started relatively recently. It helps that she also generally does not eat breakfast, so it's not too much of a stretch to skip it with her.

There are many ways to look at fasting, and though the science indicates a myriad of benefits, the best way to see if it works for you is to try it out yourself, see how your body reacts, and find a regimen that best suits your age, goals, and lifestyle.

Create your functional nutrition care plan

Knowing exactly what the best food to eat for your individual needs and goals is best achieved with the help of the experts. I've been working towards my holistic health goals with functional medicine and advanced diagnostics company LifeScience Center, and after undergoing all my tests (which I discuss in detail in Chapter 6), a personal nutrition plan was sent over to me. My personal short-term and recurring nutrition goals is to eat the best way for my upcoming sports competitions. My long-term goal, on the other hand, is to improve my cholesterol levels, protect my kidneys, and maintain a healthy weight. To give you an idea what a functional nutrition care plan can look like, I'm sharing with you mine:

John Aguilar's functional nutrition care plan

Water: Stay hydrated by drinking water to flush out toxins, help your kidneys, and stay cool during exercise
- On sedentary days – at least 2.5 litres per day
- On days with exercise – at least 500 ml for every one hour of moderate intensity and 1,000 ml for every one hour of high intensity

Cardiometabolic Food Plan
- Garlic: two to four cloves per day (may be mixed with food or consumed on its own)
- Onion: at least 1/4 bulb per day (may be mixed with food or consumed on its own)
- Chia seeds: two to three tablespoons per day (may be placed in water, milk, or mixed with rolled oats for the morning

B vitamins, especially B9 and B12, to improve neurotransmitter metabolites; have a variety of whole food and small amount of liver two to three times a week

Prebiotics and probiotics daily to improve your microbiome diversity:

- Prebiotics: vegetables and fruits in general but typically food high in fibre like asparagus, onion, banana
- Probiotics: usually found in fermented food such as yogurt, kimchi, kombucha, and sauerkraut

Food that can help improve testosterone levels

- Zinc-rich food: oysters, pumpkin seeds, eggs, cashews, nuts, legumes
- Magnesium-rich food: dark chocolate, avocado, nuts, seeds, dark green leafy vegetables
- High quality protein
- Healthy fats: avocado, nuts, seeds, fatty fish, olives, healthy oils
- Antioxidants: variety of fruits and vegetables
- Ginger

Control / Modify

- Chew slowly and thoroughly. Chewing twenty times per spoonful helps with proper digestion of food.

Others

- Follow the baking soda challenge for three consecutive days and report the result.

Baking soda challenge

The 'baking soda challenge' challenges you to drink half a glass of cold water combined with a quarter teaspoon of baking soda on an empty stomach first thing in the morning. Then it asks you to time how long it takes you to burp. If it takes longer than three to five minutes, it means you don't have enough stomach acid.

I was also provided with a weekly planner and recommended recipes to make it easier for me to find the best alternatives and work around my food sensitivities. **Note that these are all specific to my needs, which are based on laboratory results from the variety of tests that I have taken.**

Beyond looking at your own personal nutrition goals, there are nutrition strategies you can employ, depending on how you want to affect different aspects of physical performance.

Nutrition for Energy and Endurance

When we want a boost of energy, many of us know that carbohydrates are one food group we want to stock up on—hence the term 'carbo loading'. Just how much we need depends on the amount of exercise or training you put in, especially if you are entering an endurance competition. Below are some carbohydrate intake recommendations:[44]

- Moderate exercise (one hour a day): 5–7 g per kilogram of bodyweight per day
- Moderate to high-intensity exercise (one to three hours a day): 6–10 g/kg/day
- Ultra-endurance athletes (four to five hours of moderate to high-intensity exercise every day): Up to 8–12 g/kg/day

Water, naturally, is something you will need to keep up energy and endurance. Try starting with 400–800 mL/hour, and then adjust according to your thirst, sweat rate, and urine output. As a general rule, replace your fluids by 150 per cent of those you lost during your exercise, training, or high-endurance activity.

On top of carbohydrates and water, other nutrition sources also help improve endurance and energy: protein (1.4 g/kg/day; 0.3 g/kg every 3–5 hours); sodium (start initial plan at 300–600 mg/hour if you have a high sweat rate; more than 1.2 litres/hour, or if you exercise for more than for two hours); and caffeine—but this is something we will discuss further in the next part of the chapter.

Table 2.3: Different sources of protein

Eggs and Dairy	Fish and Seafood	Meat	Beans and Nuts
• Eggs: Boiled or poached ones contain 6.28 g of protein, leucine, an amino acid essential for muscle synthesis, and B vitamins. • Greek yogurt: 12–18 g of protein per 5 oz.	• Salmon and tuna: A 227-g salmon steak has 58.5 g of protein; both are a good source of omega-3 fatty acids, which prevents muscle loss in older adults.	• Chicken: Go for chicken breast and remove the skin; 120 g of this gives you 35.5 g of protein. • Turkey: One cup contains 37.23 g of protein, while a turkey drumstick has around 27 g of protein. • Fresh, lean pork: Contains 40 g of protein per cup.	• Peanuts: One cup contains around 41 g; 2 tablespoons of peanut butter, 7 g of protein; peanuts also contain 257 mg of magnesium per cup, which research[45] shows may enhance exercise performance. • Walnuts: For muscle-building, one cup of chopped, shelled walnut halves or 15.2 g of protein and 9 g of omega-3 fatty acids. • Almonds: One cup of dry roasted almonds without salt contains nearly 29 g of protein.

- Milk: For those who aren't lactose intolerant—skimmed or 1 per cent fat milk has 8 g of protein per 8 oz, while the high-protein variety contains 13 g per 8 oz; use soymilk if you are intolerant to get 7g of protein per 8 oz.

- Lean beef: Contains around 23 g of protein per 4 oz, as well as selenium, zinc, and iron, which aid in boosting energy and recovery.
- Dried beef or turkey jerky. Snack on this to get 10–15 g of protein per 8 oz.

- Edamame: Also called immature soybeans; 6 g of protein per half-cup.
- Quinoa: 9.1–15.7 g of protein per 100 g.
- Buckwheat: A seed that people can use as a grain or flour; one cup of buckwheat contains 22.5 g of protein.
- Chickpeas (aka garbanzos): 14.6 g of protein per cup; you can also take it in the form of hummus, which contains ground chickpeas, to get 7 g of protein per $1/3$ cup.
- Tofu: contains 12.68 g of protein per 100 g.
- Seeds: A half-cup of roasted sunflower seeds contains close to 14 g of protein; a half-cup of roasted pumpkin and squash seeds, 18 g.

Nutrition for Strength and Power

If you're looking to build muscle, look to food options that are good sources of protein and amino acids. Here is a quick rundown:[46]

Nutrition for Recovery

We've established in the first chapter the value of rest and recovery for peak performance—hence the need for quality sleep—and nutrition can help in that aspect, too. We identified protein as a food to build strength, but it is equally important in one's post-activity recovery, too, particularly in the thirty to forty-five-minute window that follows your exercise or training. Linus Reyes, country manager for the Philippines of Glanbia Performance Nutrition, a global company behind top sports nutrition products such as Optimum Nutrition, describes this as the **anabolic window**, wherein your muscle protein synthesis is at its highest, making it the best time for the body to absorb in the most efficient way any macronutrient you consume.

'Let's say you work out, then thirty to forty-five minutes after you consume protein. Ideally, you are in that anabolic window, then you are investing in muscle protein synthesis mode,' Linus says.

The consumption of high-quality protein also falls under 'the 4Rs framework' identified in a study of nutritional strategies surrounding post-workout recovery.[47] Below is the full framework:

- **Repair**. Ingesting high-quality protein contributes to faster tissue growth and repair.
- **Rest**. Optimizing your sleep, which we discussed at length in the first chapter.
- **Refuel**. Consuming carbohydrates for the replenishment of glycogen (stored form of glucose), and the fulfilment of one's energy requirements for tissue and immune system repair.

- **Rehydrate**. Make this a fundamental part of pre, during, and post-workout routines, to replace lost fluids and electrolytes and prevent dehydration.

To Drink or Not to Drink: Caffeine and Alcohol

Caffeine

Quickly mentioned as a performance enhancer earlier in this chapter, caffeine, for most people, has become part of people's everyday diet. Most rely on the stimulant being present in their daily cup of joe. Coffee fuels a global industry that affects a supply chain of farmers, roasters, baristas, small cafe owners, and large coffee chains, so much so that many see it as an integrated component of one's lifestyle and daily life.

Caffeine is also found naturally in tea leaves, cola nuts, guarana berries, and cacao beans, as well as in drinks other than coffee, such as sodas, and even in gums, medicines, and sports drinks. Caffeine, at low doses, has a positive effect on one's cognitive performance, memory, and brain function. Having too much caffeine, however, can contribute to elevated anxiety and nervousness[48].

According to clinical and performance nutritionist Helene Patounas of Hintsa Performance—who I initially introduced in the previous chapter—one's caffeine intake can be managed by timing when they choose to drink their coffee. Helene works with Hintsa Performance, an evidence-based coaching company that has in its roster of clients Formula 1 Champions and Fortune 500 CXOs. She helps her clients achieve peak performance, whether that's for a race or for an important business meeting or event, through proper nutrition.

'Caffeine is very well-researched as a cognitive performance enhancer, but it's about timing and not just drip-feeding caffeine into your blood the whole day, which many of us do, from habits and around the office,' Helene explains. The timing, however, varies from one person to another; so, sometimes, an F1 racer finds that taking an espresso shot would work for him right before a race, Helene says. For others, the same timing doesn't work because it causes anxiety; for others still, caffeine abstinence is key to their performance.

'People respond differently to caffeine, so practice and play with the optimal time to have [coffee],' she says. Generally, however, taking coffee close to one's bedtime is not recommended, since studies have shown that caffeine can disrupt one's sleep-wake cycle,[49] and can worsen symptoms of insomnia from those who are already suffering from it.

I have been on and off caffeine for years now, and it is a love-hate relationship depending on my body and mind's current state. I had abstained from coffee until my late thirties, just because I didn't want to be dependent on it for its benefits. I knew how some people can get cranky and just out of it if they don't have their coffee fix, so I didn't want something to have that hold on me.

But the more I discovered the benefits for both the body and mind, I decided to give it a go and true enough, it proved to be just what I needed to put my mind in the proper state every morning and prepare me not so much for the physical, but more for the mental side of the things I do.

When the pandemic set in, however, the coffee that I was consuming in the mornings started giving me palpitations, due in part to my anxiety during the time, as I was also not sleeping well and waking up very early in the morning, sometimes at 2 or 3 a.m., and not being able to sleep again. I stopped cold turkey. When the dust settled, I got back to drinking coffee, now in part to its benefits for my training, as I got back to competitive sports.

I eventually developed a very strong case of vertigo, and one of the things that my doctor did was to take me off caffeine altogether. When my vertigo cleared, coffee became a part of my routine again.

As of writing this, I'm currently off caffeine again because my vertigo has come back with a vengeance. Coffee is life, for sure, and I know its joys and benefits. I know now that it's just something that I would have to learn to live with and without for the rest of my life.

Alcohol

Ah, a totally different beast altogether. Coffee's polar opposite, but similarly used and abused. Like coffee, alcohol is another controversial drink when it comes to one's nutrition. Is alcohol consumed in moderation really good for you? When taken in moderation, some people see nothing wrong with having a glass or two a day, particularly red wine, since it has been reported to have numerous benefits. Resveratrol in particular, apart from its cardioprotective effects, also exerts anticarcinogenic, antiviral, and antioxidant properties.[50]

In Sardinia, Italy, known as one of the Blue Zones, it is normal to have one or two glasses of red wine with a meal even among those who are well into old age—which I discovered firsthand from one of the island's residents Patrizia Usala, owner of B&B Le Stanze Di Patika di Arbatax.

'Sardinian people drink a lot, and by a lot, I mean, normally, two glasses for lunch and the same for dinner,' she tells me. 'My grandfather used to say that he never saw a doctor in his life—and that the secret is to eat, every day, a piece of cheese, because we have good cheese, and a drink of wine always for breakfast, for lunch, for dinner.'

The World Health Organization, however, recently came out with a definitive guideline: No alcohol is good for the body.[51]

'Alcohol is a toxic, psychoactive, and dependence-producing substance and has been classified as a Group 1 carcinogen by the International Agency for Research on Cancer since some decades ago—this is the highest risk group, which also includes asbestos, radiation and tobacco,' the WHO states. 'Alcohol causes at least seven types of cancer, including the most common cancer types, such as bowel cancer and female breast cancer. Ethanol (alcohol) causes cancer through biological mechanisms as the compound breaks down in the body, which means that any beverage containing alcohol, regardless of its price and quality, poses a risk of developing cancer.'

It has also been said that the amount of resveratrol you would need to consume that is present in red wine would have to amount to the equivalent of a hundred to a thousand glasses to have any meaningful benefit.[52]

I myself have recently made the decision to stop drinking alcohol entirely, which for me personally, was relatively easy since I was not a heavy drinker to begin with. And the night I decided to stop drinking, I did it knowing that I would be attending a reunion with former college track teammates—in a pub, no less. I passed my own self-imposed test and managed to avoid drinking that night, and so far, I haven't had a drop again. Since then, I've noticed that my sleep and sports performance is better, and the little bump I would have in my gut when I would drink more than usual is now totally gone.

Talking to Kevin Donoghue, a Spartan pro athlete who owns multiple records in the sport, I learned that abstaining from alcohol—as well as processed food and sugar—is a major factor in what keeps him fit and healthy. In fact, he says it's the first step for anyone's fitness journey.

'It's only now that people are really starting to learn alcohol's absolute benefit to your system: None. Zero. It's a toxin. Even after a moderate night of drinking, you're so wrecked the next day that it takes you another two or three days just to recover from that one night,' says Kevin. 'So, you're always fighting this uphill battle, and then you drink again; it's the same bad cycle. I would argue the same thing about even a glass of wine. The best way to start your fitness journey is to absolutely cut out all the alcohol.'

Helene expresses the same sentiments. Living in the United Kingdom, she says that alcohol is pretty much embedded in their culture, but since curbing her own consumption following the WHO announcement, she has also experienced positive effects— better gut health, and more energy to work out.

'I think alcohol is good [when you're] in the moment, but overall, it is a stressor,' says Helene. 'You just need to consider your relationship with alcohol.'

I did a little experiment myself. After three months of zero alcohol, I decided to have a few drinks and track my body's reaction on my Oura ring. I wanted to keep as many of the variables constant. I did my usual workout and sauna session and had dinner at the usual time. Though I didn't have a hard time falling asleep and in fact was able to sleep almost immediately after I turned off the lights, my restfulness throughout the night was compromised as I woke up around 3 a.m. and was up for a significant amount of time. My HRV or heart rate variability dropped from forty to thirty milliseconds, which still falls in the normal range (20–200 milliseconds for adults)[53], but was already at the lower end of the scale. This echoes what some other people who have sleep tracking wearables tell me happens whenever they consume alcohol.

Does this mean we should all condemn and vilify alcohol consumption? Yes and no, as condemn is such a powerful word and may not be the ideal approach. Drinking, to some, is a social act, one which gives people joy and satisfaction. My wife Monica who, unlike me, continues to regularly enjoy a glass or two of wine, puts it in a very interesting light: that one glass of alcohol isn't harmful, per se, but it's also not good for you. And I say that it's interesting because Monica was diagnosed with lupus back in 2017—and one would think alcohol would be one thing that should be eliminated from her diet; but, her rheumatologist, who is helping her manage her lupus, hasn't brought it up in their consultations (unlike chips, which were specifically banned).

'[But] let me be absolutely clear: I also think alcohol does not do you any good, period. End of conversation. I also believe that, and kudos to you that you made the decision for yourself to stop drinking altogether,' Monica says to me.

We used to find joy in discovering new wines or even beer variants during our date nights and our travels, which we don't get to do now. Although I've made a clear decision to stop any alcohol consumption, I've replaced it with now trying to discover a wider range of alternatives and mocktails. So, we still go out for dinner and drinks, we just don't share the same drinks as before.

I shared this with Bobby Macasaet, who, as I mentioned earlier, went on his own transformation and went plant-based after his prostate cancer diagnosis. His advice? 'You don't have to be so dogmatic about it.' He would still on occasion have a nibble of meat even as he has gone completely plant-based.

I guess that's what I have to learn while navigating this new lifestyle change. Even as I made the decision to completely stop drinking alcohol, there's nothing wrong with sharing an occasional glass of wine with my beautiful wife on those nights when it feels just right.

Monica is also clear that she doesn't see herself making the same decision to stop drinking alcohol anytime soon, and that is something I respect. For her, drinking is not related to any physical health reasons or optimization, but rather a way for her to unwind or destress.

The other day she sends me a hilarious Instagram reel:

Child: Mommy?
Mom: Yes, sweetheart?
Child: If you didn't have wine, would you die?
Mom: I wouldn't die if I didn't have wine . . . you might though (walks away).

I'll leave it at that for now. The science is clear. The art is the conversion part, which I believe will come at some point in the future, on her own volition, and in her own good time. But for now, I'm just going with the saying 'happy wife, happy life'.

Good Nutrition: Some Tips to Remember

With all the diet trends, strategies, and information we've covered, I believe that subscribing to any particular nutritional regime is always best coupled with regular consultation with a nutritionist to see if your food choices fit your needs and your lifestyle, so you can be sure of the long-term impact on your health. (Dr Liu's research, like many innovations these days, is already leaning towards 'personalized' nutrition, she tells me). Still, while diet is subjective, there are some nutritional truths we can follow in order to optimize both our body and mind.

We've covered most of the basics—avoid ultra-processed food, increase your intake of vegetables, avoid alcohol, take caffeine only when you need it and if it suits you, and take care of your gut health. As the international authority, the World Health Organization has also laid down the ground rules when it comes to sugar, which is to have only fifty grams as one's maximum intake (taking only half of that gives you additional health benefits); salt, less than five grams of iodized salt a day; and no industrially produced trans fats (stick to healthy fats). [54]

My enriching discussions with Dr Liu and other nutrition experts also revealed these diet truths we can all abide by:

- **Banish (or at least limit) sugar and red meat**

  Even before we became informed of these practical health guidelines, many, if not all, of us grew up hearing the adage 'you are what you eat'. Dr Liu believes in this saying's powerful truth. Having had a keen interest in food since a young girl—thanks largely to her mother's delicious cooking, she tells me—Dr Liu started a career in large-scale dietary intervention trials, where she saw both the positive and harmful effects of food in animal and human nutrition. She cited working with one particular natural fatty acid called conjugated linoleic acid, which initially became popular as a weight-loss agent, until studies revealed that it caused liver damage when taken in high doses.

'It made me interested to see that you are actually what you eat, and that what we incorporate in our diets has a long-term effect on our health,' says Dr Liu.

So, for a healthy diet, we asked: What types of food should we remove? Top of Dr Liu's list is excess sugar: refined carbohydrates, sweet pastries, as well as sweetened beverages. Red meat is something she recommends people avoid, and instead recommends going for white meat or fish to fulfil their protein requirements. According to Dr Liu, a high-sugar and red-meat diet combo, especially when consumed over a long period of time, is correlated with the high risk of elevated cholesterol levels, which develop into cardiovascular diseases and Type 2 diabetes.

- **Don't be a case for bad cholesterol**
  On top of red meat, processed foods, says Dr Liu, majorly contribute to high cholesterol levels. She defines these as food with additives, such as nitrate in sausages and cured meat, as well as refined food, which loses its nutritional value in that refining process. She particularly highlights the negative health effects of consuming processed meats, which are associated with a higher risk of cardiovascular disease, Type 2 diabetes, and colon cancer.

Other risk factors for high cholesterol include age, previous history of cardiac diseases, and genetics. In my case, I have a complicated relationship with cholesterol; despite the steps I take to ensure that I remain fit and healthy, such as exercising at least five times a week and eating the right kinds of food, my 'bad' cholesterol, otherwise known as low-density lipoprotein (LDL) is elevated at twice the normal range and is considered high for prescribed limits.

To manage my cholesterol, I have already been prescribed statin therapy, or medication that lowers cholesterol levels and the risk of heart disease and stroke. It's a battle I've had for years, as I am not the most obedient when it comes to taking my statins—which, according to Dr Luis Reyes of health insurance company Maxicare, is necessary for me at this point, given that my cholesterol values have increased despite having undergone a diet and lifestyle modification. 'The most fatal thing that could happen is the cholesterol buildup in the arteries, which could lead to a heart attack,' Dr Reyes warns me.

Still, Dr Reyes also recommends that cholesterol can be managed, in terms of diet, by following the Pinggang Pinoy ('Filipino plate') guide[55], developed by the Food and Nutrition Research Institute of the Philippines' Department of Science and Technology, in collaboration with the Department of Health, the National Nutrition Council, and WHO. Generally, for a meal, half of one's plates should be allocated to fruits and vegetables, one-fourth to protein, and the rest to fibre-rich carbohydrates. There are different guidelines that you can refer to, depending on where you are in the world, making this something you can research on your own so you can choose which one resonates with you the most.

The future of food technology

One of the most interesting companies that I visited in Finland during filming my documentary series *Methods to Greatness* was Perfat Technologies, a food deep tech startup. I met the company's cofounders Jyrki Lee-Korhonen and Dr Fabio Valoppi, who introduced me to eye-opening developments that aim to make existing food healthier in light of existing consumer habits. Their innovation, using proprietary oleogel technology, is to use healthy vegetable oils (e.g. canola, sunflower, olive) and, through material physics, create an oil with the structure of solid fats so they can be used as a one-to-one replacement for the most commonly used fats, such as butter, palm oil—so food producers have an alternative, a much healthier fat that they can use in food products.

Jyrki explains further: 'The solid fats in the food industry are used because they bring structure, mouthfeel, and flavour to many processed foods. The healthy alternative would be to use liquid vegetable oils like canola oil or sunflower oil, olive oil, but they are not applicable to many foods because they're in liquid form and they don't give the structural properties that many food products require. [This is] the reason why these fats like palm oil and coconut oil are solid; they are high in saturated fats, which cause all kinds of diseases.'

Hence, 'perfect fat', Perfat's solution. The two clarify, however, that such a chemically enhanced ingredient isn't meant to take anything away from the wisdom of eating natural, whole foods.

'We don't see our food ingredient as some lab food; it is something which is produced in normal food factories. It would be used in the foods that we already consume today, and one of the things that we think is relevant to think about when you think about the healthiness of foods is that it's difficult to change people's eating habits,' Jyrki says. 'It's great to consume lots of fruit, vegetables, et cetera. But the fact is the majority of people consume foods that are processed, one way or the other.'

Their argument is that people will always consume foods such as cake and ice cream, so why not make them healthier? They let me try a cake using their 'perfect fat', and it was surprisingly good. This made me hopeful for the alternative food ingredients that food scientists not just in Finland, but from around the world, are working on and will make available for consumers in the future.

- **Rest your stomach—avoid snacking.**
  At one point in time, we've probably heard the advice to snack regularly throughout the day in order to regulate our glucose levels. According to Helene, however, recent research has revealed that giving your body a break from eating is healthier instead of constantly grazing, given that digestion is an energy-intensive process. 'And if you think about it, the kind of snacks that are available are generally ultra-processed. Sometimes these foods come in useful. You need them when you're on the run or have certain athletic pursuits, but if you look at data from different countries, snacking and ultra-processed foods are what are fuelling obesity,' Helene says.
- **Build healthy habits early in life.**
  And because of this rising global trend of childhood obesity, and the detrimental, long-term impact of red meat

and processed food consumption, both Dr Liu and Helene encourage parents to start their kids young in terms of making better food choices.

'Obesity is a big problem, because once we enter adulthood, the gradual weight gain begins, and obesity is always the strongest risk factor for a lot of things related to heart and kidney diseases, and Type 2 diabetes,' says Dr Liu. 'Provide healthy alternatives, like fruits and fresh juices, versus sweetened beverages. Swap out one thing a week, see if they like it, and gradually adapt to a healthy dietary pattern.'

The same advice is given by Helene. She says there's no better time to introduce healthy eating than early on in life, so they can develop the right nutrition habits.

- **Take note of what you eat**

  Literally, write down what you consume every day, says Dr Liu, so you can see at a glance the nutritional choices you are making—and take concrete steps to make *better* choices. 'That's such a simple task that would help you become more conscious about what you choose. When you eat a bag of chips, you write that down, and the next day you'll feel that you don't want to write it anymore, so you can remove that,' she says.

  I was also advised by LifeScience to submit a three-day photo food journal of what I eat for breakfast, lunch, dinner, and snacks. Each photo should contain all food, liquids (except water), and my levelled open palm facing up, to help approximate serving size.

- **Keep your mind in mind**

  Choose foods to help you perform at your best, since one's cognitive function also needs to be in the zone. Dr Liu recommends food from some of the oldest dietary patterns, such as extra virgin olive oil, mixed nuts, blueberries, and green leafy vegetables.

'These are the frontrunners in terms of specific food in intervals that benefit cognitive function,' says Dr Liu, who adds that these can also be found in the well-known MIND (Mediterranean-DASH Diet Intervention for Neurodegenerative Delay) diet, which is designed to aid in the health of the ageing brain. According to its guidelines, the MIND diet's list of healthy food include:[56]

- 3+ servings a day of whole grains.
- 1+ servings a day of vegetables (other than green leafy).
- 6+ servings a week of green leafy vegetables.
- 5+ servings a week of nuts.
- 4+ meals a week of beans.
- 2+ servings a week of berries.
- 2+ meals a week of poultry.
- 1+ meals a week of fish.
- Mainly olive oil if added fat is used.

The items to avoid or lessen because of their higher saturated and trans fat content are:

- Pastries and sweets with refined sugar (less than five servings a week).
- Red meat—beef, pork, lamb, and products made from these meats (less than four servings a week).
- Cheese and fried foods (less than one serving a week).
- Butter/stick margarine (less than 1 tablespoon a day).

- **Chew**

  Helene has a personal experience with a client that greatly benefited from simply chewing better. This top business executive had come to her seeking her advice to help him overcome his debilitating gut issues, for which he had already undergone major medical investigations and medication. She had him be more mindful with his eating by instructing him to chew twenty to forty times before swallowing—in six weeks, his gut health became better.

Note that mindful eating, Helene emphasizes, means really focusing on only eating; no distractions in front of you such as screens. It can be boring, she warns, but it's one simple thing you can do to help yourself eat better.

- **Hydrate with water**

  For one's daily diet, Dr Liu recommends that people drink only water in order to stay healthy. She acknowledges that this is a hard habit to form; the fact that sugar-sweetened beverages, especially soda, are so accessible and taste good makes this quite the challenge. There's also the factor of these drinks being addictive because of the presence of caffeine, as well as sugar. Research suggests that people who regularly consume sweetened beverages and then stop cold turkey experience typical cravings and withdrawal symptoms such as headaches and decreased motivation, contentment, ability to concentrate, and overall well-being[57].

Eating for Peak Performance: Race Weekend Nutrition

So, to be a top performer, what, and how, do the experts recommend we eat?

Helene shares nutrition tips that she provides to her clients—whether they're facing a Formula 1 Race, prepping for a big business meeting or presentation, or basically facing anything that requires them to be at their peak performance level. She calls it 'race weekend nutrition':

- Never try something new on performance day. If you try something new, you can get a digestive reaction, get an intolerance, or suffer from bloating. Stick to what you've tried and tested.

- Stick to a light, easily digestible meal. For example, for your everyday nutrition, it's great to consume more of the complex carbohydrates, such as unrefined grains and root vegetables. On 'race day', however, it's okay to have more refined carbs, allowing you to go for your white rice instead of brown. Don't go heavy on fats because they take longer to digest.
- Snacking isn't recommended on a daily basis, but when you need to be at your peak, make sure you're eating relatively regularly because you're burning through your blood sugar.
- Hydrate. Hydrate. Hydrate.

Taking to heart all these recommendations, tips, and pieces of advice, Helene also shares with me a beautiful sentiment about food and nutrition, which I'd like for you to take with you as you decide on your own nutritional plan: 'Food is a gift, and we need to enjoy it. I think the moment you help somebody shift their attitude to know what right foods to eat, and still give them that sense of freedom, then that is when you can see huge long-term benefits.'

My Peak Performance Diet Truths

In my personal experience, I stick to these guidelines, so to speak, so I can maintain a healthy diet as I continue on my journey towards peak performance and achieving longevity:

- **Everything in moderation**
  The pros and cons of all food and drink, except those that have been unequivocally proven by science to be bad for human consumption, will always be debated upon depending on the source. The art is really in moderate consumption.

  I've personally never been on any diet in my entire life. I've never been over or underweight and have retained my weight and general wellness and fitness since my teenage years. I've never counted calories, nor favoured any particular food group. But I've always eaten a balanced meal, and always in moderation. Yes, I would do the occasional buffet on rare occasions, but the older I got this too got tempered. Moderation, for me, is the true art of nutrition.

- **Don't go with trends**

  Always check the proponents, especially those that side on the extremes. Case in point: *The Gamechangers*—when I watched the Netflix documentary, it was so compelling and so well-made that it almost made me go vegan right then and there. It presented numerous case studies of world-class athletes and other peak performers who have embraced and have attributed their success to a plant-based diet. It presented arguments that plant-based is much more superior to consuming meat, with one study even pointing to enhanced sexual performance attributed to choosing plant-based foods as opposed to animal meat.

  But there are always two sides to a coin. Though I believe in the benefits of consuming a mostly plant-based diet, vilifying the meat and dairy industry altogether, in my opinion, is also not a sustainable way to move forward with one's message. The same can be said with the latest diet trends and most likely more to come in the future.

- **Ask for expert advice**

  Catherine Brillantes-Turvill, a close friend and owner of Nurture Wellness Village, a Filipino resort that focuses on natural healing has also pointed me in the right direction when it comes to the nutrition advice that we can best heed. As a certified educator of the Living Foods Institute, Cathy has a library of experts that she says revolutionized the way people approach nutrition. Her top recommendations are the books of Dr Andrew Weil, author of *Natural Health, Natural Medicine, Healthy Ageing: A Lifelong Guide to Your*

Well-Being, and *You Can't Afford to Get Sick: Your Optimum Health and Health Care.*

What makes Dr Weil so revolutionary, says Cathy, is that despite being a student of the conventional medicine industry, he promotes 'integrative medicine': Holistic healing that considers the body, mind, and spirit. When it comes to nutrition, specifically, he recognizes that food can function as medicine. It was an idea, says Cathy, that understandably gained him criticism in the medical field, but has since been one of the foremost authorities on how eating the right kind of natural, whole foods can help one lead a lifestyle free from the burden of disease.

Cathy distils all her learnings from Dr Weil and other top nutrition experts in her book *Turn Back Time: Natural Anti-Ageing Choices,* where she also gives a guide on achieving beauty and vitality through natural means. [58] To her, such a lifestyle is all about CHOICES:

- Choose a positive outlook. Control stress.
- Healthy eating. Hydration.
- Oxygenate through exercise, movement, and yoga qigong
- Boost your immunity with natural supplements.
- Cleanse your body, environment, and emotions.
- Embrace spa and wellness therapies.
- Do skin care, make sure to get enough sleep, and ensure social and spiritual support.

Focusing on healthy eating, Cathy shares insights on what she learned from the Living Foods Institute: primarily that a healthy diet is composed of more raw food, which, if prepared correctly, can still be as delicious as the conventional cooked, savoury meals some of us are used to. Her personal diet is ruled by a 70–30 approach—meals that are 70 per cent raw, and 30 per cent cooked, and she loads up on fresh fruits and vegetables, which she highly recommends others do, too.

My wife and our nine-year-old son paid a visit to Cathy and her husband Mike's home in the cool province of Amadeo, about an hour and a half drive from our place. Our agenda was for Cathy to show us around their local market, where we were able to purchase fresh fruits and vegetables and for her to show us how to make better food choices. Upon arriving to their house, they were also able to have our son pick fresh iceberg and romaine lettuce and plant kale seedlings in their sprawling garden farm, which is an extension of their 'Nurture Pharmacy' concept where people get to pick and take home fresh produce and are educated on how food enhances our lives beyond sustenance.

I was particularly thrilled that our son was able to pick and take home the vegetables that we would be having for the rest of the week, something that we would never be able to do back home as we just purchase our food from our neighbourhood grocery. We also took home a great tip from Cathy to keep in mind whenever we restock on groceries at home: To achieve balanced nutrition, always choose with your head, not with your heart. 'There are choices out there. Go to where there are healthy options,' Cathy says.

Supplementation

One of the biggest medical breakthroughs that have become part of our daily existence is dietary supplementation—the vitamins and minerals we take in addition to the nourishment and nutrition we get from our daily meals. Even before we enter this world, vitamins already shape our growth in the womb, as mothers are advised to consistently take their folic acid, so their babies can develop with minimal risk of birth defects. Once born, a baby's first visit to their doctor always includes a conversation on which vitamins are best to take, and that collection only grows through each life stage—especially when one is focused on optimizing their physical fitness and athleticism.

One important thing to note: In achieving one's peak performance, supplements are actually last on the list of the things you need to do. We started off this book with a focus on the importance of sleep, and for good reason—it's at the top of the list when it comes to optimal nutrition. Even if the best sources of nutrition and supplementation are within your reach, your body won't be able to function without enough sleep.

After sleep, one needs to be eating right—getting all those macronutrients from proteins, carbohydrates, and healthy fats through a well-balanced diet. We've highlighted how whole foods rich in fruits and vegetables are still key to optimizing one's health through nutrition.

Once you are fed and have rested enough, only then can you exercise and train. I've learned the repercussions of this the hard way, and I go deeper on this in the next chapter.

Fourth is hydration—replace those fluids and electrolytes that you sweat out. Do these first four things consistently, and only then would you be ready for Step 5, which is to take supplements.

According to Linus Reyes of Glanbia Performance Nutrition, this five-step philosophy is what they call the Optimum 5. Supplements are called as such, he says, and are last on the list, because their primary function is to enhance the nutrition we receive primarily through whole foods.

'A lot of companies will tell you that, "hey, you need our supplements first. You can replace your food with our supplements." We don't recommend that because you always have to get it from whole foods first,' Reyes said. 'It's human nature to try and find that quick fix, that silver bullet. They think that if they drink this tea, or drink this supplement, they'll drop the weight just like that. But it's just not true—you get out what you put in. So put in the work, and then you can start using supplements.'

Understand your supplement sources

The most common supplement most people take every day, which has been ingrained likely into our breakfast routine, is the multivitamin. Tracing back the origin of these pills, the term 'vitamin' actually came from the word 'vitamine', which is a portmanteau of 'vital amines', as coined by one of the first to formulate these—Dr Kazimierz 'Casimir' Funk. Today, these are the most common ones that we take, and we discussed them earlier as part of our micronutrient needs: Vitamins C, E, D, Zinc, and B.

What has also been recommended for my daily consumption are omega-3 fatty acid supplements, docosahexaenoic acid (DHA) and eicosapentaenoic acid (EPA). These have been identified as vital to cell health, as well as functions surrounding the heart, blood vessels, lungs, immune system, and endocrine system.[59]

Beyond these, there are countless other supplements out in the market that one may or may not take, depending on what you need and what your doctor recommends—and the options can seem endless if you don't have the proper guidance. Linus shares some practical advice on how to find the supplements that are best for you:

- Check the back label of the bottle to identify the supplements' manufacturer. Does it say 'manufactured for' or 'manufactured by'? If it's the former, be wary of the fact that these kinds of companies get their supplements from suppliers and just apply their branding, and therefore do not know the exact components of their products. On the other hand, the 'manufactured by' label means that the entire supply chain is owned by the company.
- Look at the endorsements of the supplement brand/s you are interested in—and I don't mean your online influencers. It's important that they are given a stamp of approval by

credible certification bodies, in order to demonstrate that their products are safe.

- Consumer reviews can also help, since these are feedback from actual users.
- Finally, authenticity is of utmost importance when building your supplement stack, as there are fakes out in the market that could potentially have unsafe ingredients. Check for an authenticity seal.

Supplements for sports performance

Zeroing in on supplementation for sports performance, which is what I personally need more guidance on, Linus gives me a rundown of supplements that athletes in training can consider.

He starts with essential amino acids, which usually come in the form of an energy booster that mainly has caffeine, amino acids, and electrolytes. It's a supplement that can be taken an hour before your workout.

If you are training for an ultramarathon, though, and need something to keep up your energy for longer than four hours, Linus recommends a more potent pre-workout supplement, which has more caffeine that gives you a great energy kick, as well as beta alanine, an amino acid in your body, which aids in the production of carnosine, the amino acid responsible for giving you extra endurance. It should also have L-citrulline, a vasodilator, to help open your blood vessels, and a few grams of creatine, an amino acid compound that supplies energy to the muscles.

Creatine is, to me, an old friend—it's a supplement that I have been using since my college years and, now that I am regularly training for competitions, will be part of my fitness journey again. For a sprinter like me, Glanbia's Kristine Santos confirms that creatine really is the best supplement, since I need the explosive power to run 100-metre sprints as fast as possible.

She further explains that supplementation is a routine that should be highly personalized based on an athlete's sport, workouts regimen, and lifestyle, because each different kind of athlete falls under a particular 'energy system'. For example, if you are a marathoner or a cyclist, you utilize an oxidative energy system, which is generally for low intensity, high endurance sports. Then there is the glycolytic energy system, which is more for medium to high-intensity workouts that taper and then build up to a peak—think high-intensity interval training (HIIT), dancing, thirty to forty-minute endurance sports.

I fall under the third energy system: ATP-CP, or adenosine triphosphate-creatinine phosphate. Linus says to picture ATP, which is our source of energy for use and storage at a cellular level,[60] as three tennis balls.

> 'Each time that your body will use explosive energy for movements that last for about fifteen seconds, one phosphate will convert itself into energy. So, your three phosphates, your ATP, will now be broken down into a diphosphate, because there are two left, since one phosphate became energy. What creatine does is that it brings a phosphate creatine to either replace that energy or give you more ATP stores. So, in effect when you do that fast sprint and you use a lot of ATP energy, creatine will help you recover faster, so that it gives you the effect that it gives you a stronger type of movement.'

'So, with you being a sprinter, that short amount of time that you need to finish, every second counts,' adds Kristine. 'And every bit of energy that you need to get to that twelve seconds, or even less, the creatine can help you with that.'

There is also evidence to support that creatine supplementation is good for cognitive enhancement, too, as it can help improve brain health and function, as well as memory in ageing adults.[61]

I was actually quite surprised how long creatine has been around since I was already using it back in the late nineties. More than twenty years after I last used it, creatine is now one of the most extensively studied supplements in the field of sports nutrition and exercise science. When I was using it back then, I found that it not only aided in my explosive power, but it also made me bulk up as the water retention volumizes your muscles. The danger though is that you have to make sure you drink enough water to protect your kidneys, since creatine increases water retention in muscle cells, which may lead to dehydration if you're not properly hydrated. I'm finding that with an older body, the benefits are the same, though I don't bulk up now as much as I used to.

Whey protein is also another supplement that I was taking back in the late nineties as a competitive athlete. There are many more variants available out there today—much more than what was available back in the day—and it can understandably become confusing as to which option works best. Linus helps me out by explaining first the difference between variants with whey protein isolates and those with whey protein concentrate. 'Whey protein isolates are a highly refined form of whey protein, containing a higher percentage of protein by concentration compared to whey protein concentrate,' he says. Some variants with whey protein isolates are also mixed with BCAAs (branched-chain amino acids), making it an ideal choice for individuals looking to increase their protein intake without excess carbs and fats.

For those seeking a leaner option with even fewer carbohydrates, fats, and cholesterol, variants that contain whey protein isolates with protein concentrations of 90 per cent above are their best bet. They are suitable for individuals focused on weight management or strict macronutrient counting, as well as athletes preparing for competitions—particularly those aiming to cut weight while maintaining muscle mass.

Linus notes, however, that it is important to consider individual needs and preferences when choosing between whey protein concentrate and whey protein isolate. Whey protein isolate, being pre-digested and broken down into smaller peptides, offers faster and more efficient absorption, making it ideal for post-workout consumption during the anabolic window. On the other hand, whey protein concentrate provides a broader spectrum of nutrients and may be preferred by some individuals for its taste and texture.

Beyond whey protein, alternative options are available, Linus tells me, such as plant-based proteins for vegetarians, vegans, or those with lactose intolerance. Plant proteins, derived from sources like peas and rice, offer a viable alternative for individuals seeking protein supplementation without animal-derived ingredients. Additionally, for those looking for slow-digesting proteins suitable for nighttime consumption or intermittent fasting, casein protein presents an excellent option. Casein protein, with its prolonged digestion period of four to eight hours, supports muscle repair and growth during periods of rest, making it an ideal choice for overnight supplementation or fasting periods.

Herbal supplements for sports performance

Herbal supplements have also claimed significant shelf space in many health stores and pharmacies, and for good reason—before the advent of modern science, herbs have traditionally been used as medicine. Research has shown that these supplements can enhance one's physical performance: [62]

- Capsaicin: Comes from capsicum such as cayenne, red, and chili peppers, and has been classified by the United States Pharmacopeia as a stimulant.
- Ginkgo biloba: The Gingko biloba leaf extract comes from the Chinese Ginkgo tree, which has been around for two hundred million years, and is believed to improve blood circulation and exercise performance.
- Ginseng: Belongs to the plant family Araliaceae. Has anti-stress effects, and ideally helps athletes undergo more intense training, combat fatigue, and, during competition, increase stamina.

- Kava kava and St. John's wort: Kava kava, is the peeled and dried root of a South Pacific herb called *Piper methysticum* G. Forster, which traditionally has been used as a ritual beverage because of its calming properties. St. John's wort comes from the dried parts of *Hypericum perforatum* and is primarily used as an antidepressant. Both are thought to reduce anxiety in athletes that may disrupt their sport performance.

Supplements for cognitive performance

While I dedicate a later chapter to optimizing one's mind, it's worth noting here some supplements that have been identified as 'cognitive enhancers'. To perform at your best, whether that's for sports or any just on a daily basis, there is research that suggests that omega-3 fatty acids and nootropics and adaptogens are the best supplements for the mind.

Studies on omega-3 fatty acids, which again include DHA and EPA, have demonstrated their cognitive-enhancing abilities across all ages, as these are essential components of our nerve cell membranes.[63] Deficiency of these also show detrimental effects on brain development, and, in your older years, lead to cognitive impairment, which can lead to neurodegenerative disorders.

Nootropics, or 'smart drugs', are substances that are classified as such because of their ability to 'improve the brain's supply of glucose and oxygen, have antihypoxic effects, and protect brain tissue from neurotoxicity'.[64] Adaptogens, on the other hand come from plants and mushrooms and help the body deal with stress, anxiety, and fatigue in the short term.[65] Some of the herbal supplements mentioned earlier, such as gingko biloba and ginseng, also fall under this group, while some nootropics need a prescription.[66]

Supplements for longevity

The Maximon Longevity Compendium: A Practical Guide to Extending Your Healthy Lifespan, dedicates a section to supplements that support one's health as one ages. Below is a snapshot of these supplements, and how these address particular health concerns:

Supplements for rest

Neuroscientist Dr Andrew Huberman recommends this 'sleep stack' when it comes to supplementation, which he says many people have reported can make them feel very drowsy, helps them get into deep sleep, and makes them feel refreshed with no grogginess upon waking[67]:

- Magnesium threonate, 145 mg: Some people report that this upsets their gut, and if this happens to you, stop it immediately, says Huberman.
- Apigenin, 50 mg.
- Theonin, 100–400 mg.

Huberman makes a note, however, that it is not necessary to take all three, or even one of these supplements, if you are able to sleep without any issues; and that if you do decide to take one, two, or all of these, to first reach out to your physician and consult with them. He does emphasize that the margin of safety of these three supplements is quite broad—but again, err on the side of safety and talk to your doctor first.

DHA and EPA have also been reported to improve sleep quality, especially for middle to old-age adults who have difficulty sleeping.[68]

This is something that I myself take nightly, around thirty minutes before bedtime. I have been taking these more as a recommendation of my nutritionist and not necessarily to improve my sleep quality, but if it helps improve my sleep, that would be an added benefit I would gladly take but not necessarily attribute a good night's sleep to.

On nights that I feel I really need help, I take melatonin but use this only on very rare occasions when I know that I won't be able to calm my mind and will have a hard time settling my thoughts.

My Supplement Protocol

Based on my care plan by LifeScience, I was given the following supplement protocol based on my specific needs and goals:

1. Essential Multivitamins
2. Omega-3 Fish Oil 720 EPA-DHA
3. NAC (N-Acetyl-Cysteine)
4. Multi-Strain Probiotic Blend

I also, through my personal experience and research, take the following supplements to aid in sports performance:

1. Whey Protein
2. Creatine
3. BCAAs
4. Collagen

It is my hope that armed with all this information about supplementation, you can approach your nutritionist with the right questions as to which ones will best work for you, so you can take home your own protocol and enrich your nutrition and supplementation in a safe, effective, and healthy way.

Table 2.4: A guide to using supplements

Supplement	Daily dose	What it does	How it could help you	Risks
NAD+ Nicotinamide adenine dinucleotide, a coenzyme that naturally occurs in the cells of all living organisms, from fruit flies to humans.	250 mg–1 g (especially on exercise days).	Helps convert nutrients from food into energy. Plays a crucial role in maintaining DNA health and regulating cellular functions. Needed by specific enzymes in cells such as sirtuins, which protect DNA from damage by environmental factors such as pollution, unhealthy diet, and smoking.	Prevents cancer and as cognitive and neurodegenerative diseases. Vital to the proper functioning of the immune system.	Those with existing or cured cancer or has a family history of cancer (can exacerbate tumours). Those with asthma or other immune diseases should consult first with their doctor.

	Dosage	Mechanism	Benefits	Cautions
Resveratrol A polyphenol produced by plants and found in a variety of foods, including peanuts, blueberries, and raspberries, as well as red wine (but only in very small traces).	250–500 mg	A powerful antioxidant neutralizing free radicals and preventing them from damaging our cells and the inner walls of arteries. At the molecular level, an activator of Sirtuin 1, a tumour suppressor and DNA repair protein.	Reported to help in protecting the heart, and preventing respiratory, neurodegenerative, and metabolic diseases, as well as diabetes, inflammation, joint pain, and skin ageing.	Consult with your doctor if you: Have a bleeding disorder Take blood-thinning drugs, blood pressure drugs, cancer treatments, MAOI antidepressants, antivirals, antifungals, NSAID painkillers, and supplements such as St. John's wort, garlic, and ginkgo regularly.
Pterostilbene A polyphenol found in blueberries, nuts, and grapes. A potent antioxidant, with a structure that is comparable to resveratrol but is more easily absorbed by one's cells.	50–250 mg	Helps in the production of NAD+ molecules, upregulates a variety of mitochondrial genes and helps in cellular energy production.	Data shows anti-inflammatory effects.	

Coenzyme Q10 A powerful antioxidant.	30–300 mg	Occurs naturally in the body in the form of ubiquinol. Protects mitochondrial and lipid membranes from free radicals.	Is an essential part of the electron transport chain (ETC) reaction, which leads to the production of energy within mitochondria and our cells. Improves heart health, reproduction, brain health, energy levels, anti-ageing, eyesight improvement, immune system support, reduced inflammation, firmer skin, free radical damage protection.	No significant side effects; consult with doctor if any are experienced.
Apigenin A natural flavonoid compound present in vegetables such as celery, fruits such as oranges, and herbs such as chamomile, parsley, thyme, oregano, and basil.	20–50 mg	Studies show that apigenin inhibits CD38, one of the main NAD+ degrading enzymes in human tissues, including the liver, brain, heart, and kidney. CD38 levels increase in several tissues during ageing.	CD38 inhibition by apigenin increases the intracellular NAD+ levels and improves several aspects of glucose and lipid Homeostasis.	Higher doses can cause stomach discomfort.

	Dosage			
Betaine AKA trimethylglycine (TMG), a molecule naturally present in the body. Involved in liver function and cellular reproduction.	500 mg–6 g (betaine powder) 650 mg–2 g (betaine-HCl)	Provides additional methyl groups needed in various cellular methylation processes—many important biomolecules such as CoQ10, melatonin, serotonin, and glutathione depend on methylation.	Has shown some interesting effects by itself on cardiovascular and metabolic disease.	Higher doses can cause stomach issues such as indigestion, nausea, bloating, vomiting, diarrhoea, and cramps. In rare cases, it could increase the amount of methionine (amino acid) significantly, which could cause fluid build-up around the brain.
EGCG (Epigallocatechin-3-gallate) A potent antioxidant which can help reduce bad cholesterol (LDL) levels. Traces of EGCG are found in green tea, matcha tea, strawberries, cherries, avocados, pistachio, and hazelnuts.	250–400 mg	Promotes the formation and maintenance of the synaptic connections between neurons, which is helpful for good memory and learning abilities. Protects cells from damage caused by oxidative stress and suppresses the activity of pro inflammatory chemicals produced in the body.	Diminishes the risk of developing Alzheimer's disease.	Overdosing at more than 800 mg per day could damage the liver and kidneys. Not for those with fatty liver disease.

Collagen The most abundant protein in the body—'the glue that holds the body together'	2–10 g of hydrolyzed collagen peptides.	The main component of the extracellular matrix (outside of cells), and is present in many tissues such as muscles, blood vessels, the digestive system, and the skin.	Can recycle your damaged extracellular matrix and improve its functionality. Improves bone health by preventing bone loss and joint pain, reduces inflammation, and improves heart and brain functions. Optimum collagen levels help skin cells to rejuvenate and repair any damages.	Some people may show allergic reactions to collagen supplements from animal sources, as most collagen products are animal-based.
Chondroitin Chondroitin-sulphate is a glycosaminoglycan attached to proteins in the extracellular matrix and is naturally produced by the body.	800–1200 mg	Can reverse the decline of collagen, laminin, integrin, and elastic fibre molecules brought about by ageing, and help in maintaining extracellular matrix homeostasis.	Inhibits chronic inflammation and prevents cancer. Improves all causes of mortality, overall health, and skin longevity. Used for osteoarthritis and cataracts.	Not for asthma and prostate cancer patients. Other possible side effects include stomach pain, nausea, and diarrhoea.

AKG (alpha-ketoglutarate) A small molecule that is naturally occurring in the body and is involved in numerous metabolic and cellular pathways.	Up to 2 g	Works as an energy donor, a precursor in amino acid production, and cellular signalling molecule.	Works in various pathways in our body, to help build muscle and heal wounds—popular among bodybuilders. Evidence shows that AKG can influence ageing, reduce age-related frailty, and increase lifespan.	No significant side effects; consult with doctor if any are experienced.
Senolytics: **Fisetin** (found in many plants such as legume families, the parrot tree, and in small amounts in strawberries). **Quercetin** (a natural pigment found in chilies, red onions, capers, and some berries).	Should be administered intermittently, for a few days every other week or once a month.	Fisetin is an excellent antioxidant polyphenol and effective in eliminating senescent or 'zombie' cells, or cells that do not enter their programmed death cycle and stay active in a state called cellular senescence. Quercetin is one of the most active flavonoids with strong senolytic benefits.	Reinforces the immune system, which, while designed to find and clean out zombie cells, weaken with age. Some known senolytic compounds are repurposed anti-cancer molecules (such as the chemotherapeutic drug dasatinib).	No significant side effects; consult with doctor if any are experienced.

Your to-do list to achieve peak nutrition:

- **Re-evaluate your daily diet.** Make a list of all the food you eat, if you are getting the right amount of macro and micronutrients, and see what you need to add, lessen, eliminate from your diet to improve your nutrition.
- **Check in with your nutritionist.** Create a list of fitness goals and build a nutrition plan with him/her and explore a supplementation plan as well based on your targets.
- **Visit your local farmer's market.** Discover all the fruits and vegetables available and add a couple of new ones to your daily diet.
- **Take a break from alcohol and see how it goes.** Try to see how you do at your next social activity without drinking—or, if you're the host, serving—alcohol. It might even be fun to see how many ways you can creatively come up with alternatives if you really put your mind to it.

Chapter 3

Movement, Exercise, Training

Sardinia, Italy. In this part of the world, known as a Blue Zone, a region where people are known to live longer, healthier lives compared to the global average, it is not surprising to see the elderly—think over eighty—still navigating four flights of stairs to reach their home, all while carrying a heavy bucket of water. Just ask Patrizia Usala, owner of the bed and breakfast Le Stanze Di Patika di Arbatax, as her eighty-six-year-old father is someone who is able to accomplish such a task without any assistance. Keeping active in retirement age is but one of the 'secrets' of longevity in Sardinia, Patrizia tells me, where people find value in working the earth.

'We like to say that fields are our "natural gyms",' Patrizia says.

Exercise, to Sardinians, does not need to be a workout regime that many of us see as an add-on to our daily activities. To them, exercise is integrated into their daily tasks—housework, gardening, and running errands. They also prefer to walk, Patrizia says, and the mountainous terrain naturally lets them get those daily steps in.

And that's what movement should ideally be to all of us: Natural and integrated, something that's part of our everyday existence.

For some people such as myself, movement is not something that my urban environment naturally predisposes me to, and so that is why I make sure I make time for regular exercise and make it part of my life and lifestyle.

Unlike the Sardinians, I live in urban Manila, where, unfortunately, cars are the default mode of transportation. Ours is not a walkable city, we get our water on tap, and the turf grass I've installed in our backyard doesn't allow for much gardening either.

But despite the lack of movement as a natural function of the life I lead, I remember the exact moment when I decided to make movement an integral part of it. I was about nine years old, on top of our house's gate which I had just climbed at the end of a long day playing video games at our next-door neighbour's house. I remember a brief pause, just as I was about to jump into our garage, thinking to myself and realizing that I had spent the entire day in front of a screen playing a game that, at the end of the day, I had nothing to show for. I felt lethargic and, quite frankly, sick. I had just had a profound realization and swore I would do something more productive the next day and actually move my body instead of just 'wasting away' my time and my day staring at a screen. I was nine years old!

Motivation to Move

Little did I know back then, but that moment planted a seed and initial aspiration for me to become an athlete. I did not have a specific sport in mind per se, but I wanted to always be out doing something—biking, running around and exploring our village. My father would eventually take me with him when he started playing tennis, and that began my initial foray into competitive sports and training.

Not everyone is cut out or aspires to be an athlete, but, like the residents of Sardinia, such as Patrizia and their famed centenarians, it is ideal that we strive to incorporate movement in everything we do. It might not be automatic, given today's modern world and lifestyle, where we don't need to herd sheep and fetch our water from a well or, for some people, to not even have walkable or bikeable roads to get to work or places of leisure, but I believe it's just a matter of finding your motivation to move.

Take, for example, two-time Southeast Asian Games marathoner Jasmine Goh, a Singaporean who started 'late' in her running career at the age of thirty-two back in 2011. Her motivation at the time, coming out of a divorce, was to become a strong role model for her two daughters.

'I wanted them to see that Mommy's empowered by the circumstances [at the time], that we are not victims of those circumstances,' Jasmine says. 'I can't change a lot of things, but I can make them see that I'm getting my life in order.'

Movement, specifically, running, became Jasmine's refuge, so she could first take charge of her physical health, so that, in her words, she could start filling her cup so she could have a full cup to give. It's not like she had never exercised, but Jasmine admitted struggling previously to stick to her resolve to be active—that, and she was a stay-at-home mom busy raising her children.

'So, imagine a stay-at-home mom who has never gone shopping, always stayed at home for almost four years of her life,' Jasmine recalls. 'There was not a lot of social media then; I was not really going out or taking care of myself.'

Running gave her focus, and soon, Jasmine cemented her commitment to it by signing up for a marathon when she found an opportunity—and the rest, as they say, is history.

Today, this extraordinary marathoner credits her mental resilience to her running journey, allowing her to thrive as a mother, an athlete, and as a businesswoman at the helm of innovation strategy firm, Asia Innovate Hub, in Singapore.

'If you can change yourself physically, what is so difficult about everything else? I have this strong belief that anyone can transform. You can transform anything, as soon as the goal resonates with you,' Jasmine says.

It's also not surprising how Jasmine is able to lead such an active lifestyle and able to train, since Singapore is now considered as having elements that Blue Zones across the world share. National

Geographic journalist and author Dan Buettner in his Netflix documentary series *Live to 100: Secrets of the Blue Zones*, points to the existence of public health facilities in Singapore that people have access to.

As a frequent visitor to Singapore, I've seen exactly how one can be encouraged to move. Since most people rely on public transportation, walking, despite the heat, is always an option. There are also many parks and open spaces where one can run, bike, or just spend time in nature, within this small 'garden city'.

In Loma Linda, a Blue Zone known to have exceptional exercise facilities for the elderly, I was truly impressed with how the Loma Linda University's Drayson Center gym offered such a wide variety of exercise, sports, recreation, and social activities to its members. It has everything in terms of facilities, but most noteworthy were the senior classes specifically for the elderly.

During my visit, I saw a group of seniors doing low-impact cardio in the pool. They all looked like they were having a great time, and I wouldn't be surprised if they also spent time socially outside of these classes.

The Movement, Exercise, and Training Journey

In this chapter, I focus on three key terms: movement, exercise, and training. They may seem interchangeable, but each represents distinct concepts within the realm of physical activity and fitness— Jasmine's story demonstrates best the progression across these three, as one creates more structure and develops specific goals surrounding physical fitness. These three, essentially, describe a journey, and the destination varies from person to person.

So, before we dive deep into the importance of each, let's do a rundown of their nuances:

Movement

- Encompasses all forms of physical activity, whether purposeful or incidental, and includes activities of daily living such as walking, standing, bending, and reaching.
- Is fundamental to human function and is essential for maintaining mobility, flexibility, and overall health.
- Examples are walking to and from work, going up the stairs, housework.

Exercise

- A subset of movement that involves planned, structured, and repetitive physical activity with the specific goal of improving or maintaining physical fitness.
- Typically performed with the intention of achieving health-related outcomes, such as cardiovascular fitness, muscular strength, endurance, flexibility, or body composition.
- Are designed with specific parameters, which include intensity, duration, frequency, and type of activity—all tailored to one's individual goals and fitness levels.
- Examples are running, going the gym, swimming, biking.

Training

- Goes beyond simple exercise and involves a systematic and progressive approach designed to enhance athletic performance, aimed at achieving specific performance goals and competitive outcomes.
- Incorporate principles of periodization, progression, and specificity to optimize adaptation and performance gains over time.
- Geared towards achieving targeted improvements in performance, whether in sports, fitness competitions, or specific physical pursuits.

- Examples are training for a marathon, triathlon, competitive team sports.

In a nutshell, movement is found in all daily physical activities, which includes exercise and training—with the latter two having more structure and geared toward specific health or sports competition goals. While they are all related concepts, understanding their distinctions can help you customize your approach to physical activity based on personal goals, preferences, lifestyle, and fitness levels.

From Movement to Exercise

Exercise, ideally, should be part of our everyday routine. It's something that we should like, if not enjoy, doing. Depending on your daily activities, Matti Kontsas, coaching director and senior performance coach at Hintsa Performance, also believes that people should first understand what kind of movement they enjoy doing, so they can motivate themselves to get started.

'I feel like people overcomplicate it in the sense of, am I doing enough for it to be beneficial? I feel like that's a silly question because you've got to get to a place where you do something so that you can build on that something,' Matti says.

For him, the first thing to look at when deciding on the kind of exercise you'd like to do, if you don't have a routine down pat yet, is to understand how it fits into your life—is it a social activity for you, or something you'd rather do alone?

Once you have the answer to that, identify how you can start small with your exercise, so you can form a daily healthy habit, and continue to build on your routine from there. If you want to run, don't plan on achieving ten kilometres right away, as you will probably lose your motivation quickly. Instead, go for more achievable goals, such as one kilometre a day three times a week. Soon you'll see that you're able to run two, three kilometres, until you finally reach your goal.

Imperfection, when it comes to building exercise routines, is also part of enjoying one's exercise, says Matti. You can get expert advice on a personal exercise plan that fits you best, which is great, but if you're starting from step 1, you don't have to follow it rigidly—figure out what you can do at the moment, and simply build on that progression.

When I retired from competitive sports in my early twenties, I decided that I would no longer compete but would continue to exercise as part of my lifestyle. I genuinely enjoy exercising regardless of the sport. Going to the gym, running, cycling, swimming, golf. All of these sports I truly enjoy. I also prefer sports that allow me the flexibility to do them anytime and can fit into my schedule. With the exception of golf, which I prefer to play with other people if I have a chance, most of the sports I engage in can be played alone at my own pace and at my own time and convenience.

Some people need or look for the social component and are also more motivated when they engage in team sports or have someone—a training partner or teammate—they are accountable to. It's important to know your preference so you can make sure you are motivating yourself or are being motivated by others the right way.

From Exercise to Training

Exercise helps us attain our general fitness goals, which enable us to maintain our health, ideally, for a long period of time. This was my motivation for exercising all these years. I was exercising because I wanted to look good, feel good, and be able to actively engage in sports for the sheer enjoyment of it.

However, there came a point when I was starting to miss the thrill of competition. Competition, and the training that comes with it, engages you in so many more ways that merely exercising just for health reasons cannot. I found that through the years, I would find sports that I would want to excel in and start training for. It started with joining ten-kilometre runs, and eventually obstacle races such as the Spartan Race and Ninja Obstacle Course Races.

It was good for the soul to participate in these sports for recreation, but I wanted more.

Training for competition

The decision to get back to competitive sprinting came when I saw an announcement on social media on the upcoming Philippine Masters Athletics Championships. Masters is the category for athletes aged thirty-five and above. The winners in each event, where you compete with other master athletes in your age category (mine was the forty-five to forty-nine age group), would get to represent the country in the Asian Masters Athletics Championships. I finally had a goal, and I wanted the thrill of competition so bad.

I also felt that this was my second chance. Although I had broken multiple track and field records as a high school and collegiate athlete and represented the country in a few international competitions, I had missed the opportunity to be a regular member of the national team. I had made a decision to retire from my sport in my early twenties so I could pursue a career, and eventually, run my own business. If I was making a comeback, I wanted to make sure that I was finally representing the country as a bona fide member of Team Philippines.

Fitness was not the issue when I decided to train for my favourite event, the 100-metre dash. The issue was that it had been many years since I had run a full-out sprint. As any parent, who, at one point in their lives had to sprint after their young toddler who decided to veer ever so slightly towards an oncoming bike/car/ anything that is bigger and could potentially maim or kill their child, I, too, had experienced the sudden burst of adrenaline that allowed one to reach extraordinary speeds. It's what happens to our back/ hamstrings/other vulnerable middle-aged body parts right after that makes us realize that hey, we are no longer spring chickens.

To train for the competition, I knew I had to train in a proper track oval. I had decided to return to my old stomping grounds and joined the track training of my alma mater, the Ateneo de Manila University. I must admit I felt a bit uneasy when I first stepped on the track oval on my first day of training, running with college kids less than half my age. 'Wow, you're as old as my dad!' one student exclaimed when he found out how old I was. I took it as a compliment.

For the next few months, I would train specifically for my favourite event, the 100-metre dash. My training would ideally be highly targeted and specific, as my body would be trained to respond to the speed and power training required to do well in the event.

Getting specific

As a sprinter, I took time to consult with Europe-based professional strength and conditioning Coach Carlo Buzzichelli, director of the ISCI or the International Strength and Conditioning Institute. His impressive portfolio includes collaborations with Olympic athletes and national record holders, showcasing his proficiency in sculpting the careers of elite performers.

Coach Carlo shared with me insights into his specialized field, particularly focusing on my sport and event, sprinting. In the world of athletics, especially in the realm of sprinting, Coach Carlo says achieving peak performance demands a nuanced approach to training. For me, for example, a forty-five-year-old sprinter seeking to recapture the speed of my youth, it begins with a deep understanding of my unique physiological makeup. Having a slower recovery rate and myriad external commitments, I have to deal with a different set of challenges compared to my younger counterparts.

The cornerstone of Coach Carlo's approach in building specific training regimens lies in identifying the factors hindering performance. That's the beauty of working with a coach—you undergo comprehensive assessments and keen observation, and along the way, uncover areas ripe for improvement, be it in explosive strength or neuromuscular coordination—or in my case, the challenges of a busy life. From there, you can tailor training regimens to mimic the demands of the activity you are training for, so that every aspect of your programme, from power tests to drill execution, is meticulously designed to enhance your proficiency.

Throughout the training process, Coach Carlo emphasizes the importance of consistency, patience, and attention to detail. While achieving significant performance improvements may require time and effort, Coach Carlo believes in the power of incremental gains accumulated through focused and disciplined training. By remaining committed to the process and maintaining a growth mindset, athletes can unlock their full potential and achieve their desired outcomes.

There is also the fundamental principle of overload, or the gradual progression towards peak performance. Coach Carlo emphasizes in our conversation the importance of addressing imbalances and weaknesses, followed by systematic strength and power development. Each phase of the training cycle, meticulously structured over weeks, aims to push the boundaries of the athlete's capabilities without risking overexertion.

And that is a balance that you need to strike in your training: progression and recovery. Push yourself to your limits, yes, but also allow sufficient time for adaptation and rejuvenation, Coach Carlo advises.

For years, I've been exercising and 'training' without actually having a clear goal in mind. If you take a look at your current exercise or training regimen, are you on a path towards improvement and progression? Or do you find yourself on a never-ending plateau?

My training regimen

Upon sharing with Coach Carlo my ambition of revitalizing my sprinting career, he started me off with a meticulous assessment of my baseline capabilities through a series of power tests, which measures explosive strength, and a reactive strength index test, which assesses the ability to utilize elastic energy. These evaluations unearthed valuable insights into my explosive strength and reactive capabilities, laying the foundation for targeted interventions.

I was pretty proud of his assessment: 'Your explosive strength is pretty good: way above average, for an athlete of your age. Of course, you expect a master sprinter to be explosive, nevertheless, it is a very good starting point.' He then turned his focus on my neuromuscular characteristics and found room for improvement in the elastic reactive component. He delves into the technical aspect of sprinting, highlighting my tendency to plantar flex during drills. He stresses the importance of dorsiflexion in sprinting drills, signalling a crucial aspect for me to address.

I must admit I was a bit hopeful of how he would assess my physicality. I was proud of the work I've put in all these years and to hear him say that I still had the explosive strength was the validation I needed to have the confidence to take things to the next level.

He then gave me an outline of a comprehensive strategy aimed at optimizing my strength and conditioning:

- Focus on addressing muscular imbalance in the first four weeks of training.
- Increase joint strength in weeks five to ten.
- Maximize power in weeks eleven to twelve.
- Taper training in the last two weeks before competition.
- Work on improving elastic component and reactive strength.
- Monitor development of reactive strength index over time.
- Optimize aspects like nutrition and recovery.

Coach Carlo's expertise spans across various sports, but his passion lies in track and field, particularly the 100-metre sprint. I believe this is arguably the most coveted event in track and field, because the one who finishes first is declared the fastest man or woman of the game. It is sport in its purest form. The event does not care how much experience, training, pedigree, or skill you have. It merely declares the winner as the first person who gets from point A to point B in the fastest time possible.

Coach Carlo emphasized to me the importance of having a systematic tracking of training variables, namely **volume**, **intensity**, and **frequency**. These variables, he says, serve as crucial metrics in designing personalized training programmes tailored to each athlete's needs and goals. By meticulously monitoring and adjusting these parameters, coaches can optimize the effectiveness of training regimens while minimizing the risk of overtraining and injury.

He also highlighted how having a balanced training programme addresses the specific needs of older athletes such as myself, and to consider not only physical conditioning, but also nutritional support and recovery strategies to maximize performance gains.

I also consulted with US-based track and field coach and trainer Gary Cablayan, who gave me his recommendations based on my current training regimen and schedule. He initially recommended doing track workouts on Mondays, Wednesdays, and Saturdays, focused on sprinting, with specific drills and exercises tailored to improve speed and technique. My weight training sessions with Coach Carlo would therefore be scheduled on Tuesdays, Thursdays, and Fridays, with plyometric exercises integrated into my regimen to enhance explosive strength and improve sprinting performance.

Between plyometric sessions and track workouts, it's important to recover properly, he reminds me, to prevent overtraining. The plan we are working on will, therefore, prioritize flexibility and recovery work so I can avoid injury, with easy days scheduled on Tuesdays and Fridays for active recovery, mobility work, and light exercises to flush out muscles.

Sunday is my designated rest day in the training schedule.

Overall, the training regimen prescribed by Coach Gary and Coach Carlo aims to optimize my performance as a sprinter while ensuring safety, health, and well-being throughout the process.

The plan is structured yet flexible, with a focus on gradual progression and continuous improvement.

It seemed like the perfect plan from the start. After the first week of doing both programmes from both coaches, I was fine. By the second week, my body reminded me that I was already forty-five.

To cut a long story short, I ended up combining the programme of both coaches, overworked my body, and strained my hamstrings in the process. We then adjusted the programme, significantly reducing the load and increasing the number of my recovery days. It was Coach Gary who then gave me the advice to just always listen to my body. From that point onwards, I have made sure to always listen to how my body feels, regardless of the workout for that day. I would then adjust the load and intensity accordingly.

I managed to finish second in the 100-metre dash in the Philippine Masters Athletics Championships, which earned me a slot in the national team for the Asian Masters Athletics Championships. I would go on to anchor our team there to a silver medal finish in the 4x100 metres relay behind sprint superpower Japan. The following year, I eventually won the 100-metre dash gold at the Philippine Masters Athletics Championships. As of this book's writing, I had just come back from competing at the 25th World Masters Athletics Championships in Gothenburg, Sweden. It was a memorable championship as I had the honour of carrying our country's flag during the parade of athletes. Though I did not win any medals, I had the opportunity to go head-to-head against former Olympians and European champions.

I have every intention of continuing to perform at this level for years to come. What I realize however, is that my coaches can only support me so much, as I have to constantly communicate to them how my body is responding to the training and recovery protocols. To do so, listening to my body and following my instincts will take on a whole new level of importance.

The routines and habits needed to train and achieve peak performance are already there. But this ability, however, did not come overnight. It's something that I attribute to being given exposure to sports from an early age.

Starting Them Young

Like many athletes, the regimen, routines, and ability to take instruction and coaching usually starts at a young age. I was around eleven when my father introduced me to tennis, a sport that he was religiously playing at the time. It started innocently enough, as I would just tag along and hit a few balls in between the games he would play with his buddies. He eventually got a professional to teach me the basics, and I got hooked.

For the next few years, I would train in various tennis clinics with different coaches and would compete in a number of tournaments. By joining these tournaments, I realized a number of things. First, kids who were really exceptional started learning the sport much younger. They started playing at around six or seven years old and were way better skill-wise than I was.

I also had a weakness that would make it difficult for me to win: I was erratic and had a very unreliable second serve. I had the tendency to want to finish the point soon and blast away my groundstrokes and my serve. The point would usually end with me making an unforced error or double faulting.

Though I never won any of the tournaments I joined, training for them allowed me to shape early habits. Putting in hours of training under the sun and getting used to the repetition and constant movement, served as a solid foundation for my future success as a track athlete.

When I eventually tried out for my high school's track team during my sophomore year, I was instantly the fastest recruit. I was a natural at sprinting, with my explosive speed and propensity for power over endurance. I quit tennis altogether as I had found a new sport, a sport that I was perfectly suited for. In the next few years, I would dominate my events and set new records in the 100-metre dash, pole vault, and the decathlon.

I also learned a valuable lesson: it's okay to quit and do something else you're better suited for. I was not getting the results as a tennis player but was able to find success and fulfilment in another sport. The medals that I won and the records that I broke were a direct result of working hard at something I was good at and making sure that I put in the time and effort. It was a life lesson that I take with me to this day and has informed my approach to accomplishing my goals.

Speaking of medals, I'll go ahead and say it: back in the day, the only people who got medals were those who came in first, second, or third. Call me old-fashioned, but I'm part of those who don't think medals should be given to anyone who crosses the finish line or finishes a race.

These days, for most races, there's a medal waiting for you at the finish line, regardless of if you came first or last. A finisher's medal to me is a modern-day construct that allows people to have a memento of the moment, losing its original lustre that symbolizes triumph over your competitors. It's become the perfect social proof on social media. Everybody who finishes the race brandishes their medal, preferably in front of the finish line. I, myself, have been guilty of this for most races that I've joined since the 2010's.

When my then seven-year-old son crossed the finish line for his first-ever Spartan Kids race, he was pale as a ghost. Like most of the other kids' parents, I had shadowed him the entire 1.5-kilometre obstacle race, egging him on for every obstacle and shouting, 'Let's go David!' and 'Faster! You can pass the next kid!' The balancing act of allowing him to have fun but also trying to instill a competitive spirit is, I have to admit, quite difficult.

When he received his finisher's medal at the finish line and we posed for pictures after, a few things were going through my mind. What did this experience teach him? Even if he did not technically 'win' the race, will this motivate him to try harder or will it make this experience irrelevant since he received a medal anyway?

As we made our way back home, I snuck a look back at him in the back seat, he was there plastered and sound asleep. Why was I overthinking this? My boy just finished his first Spartan Kids race and I couldn't be prouder. That's all that matters for now.

I wondered after that race if my thoughts were even valid or if I was just being too hard on my expectations for the life lessons he should have learned from the experience. In my conversation with Scott Larsen, coach and founder of Tri Edge Team Triathlon Coaching in Singapore, he tells me that parents face challenges exposing children to sports due to time and access issues, but parents should let children choose their own sports to avoid burnout and ensure intrinsic motivation.

When I asked him for advice on how to support my son's self-discovery through various sports without forcing a specific interest, he said, 'Prioritize the child's interests and potential over personal desires. Fathers and mothers can foster their children's athletic development by exposing them to various sports and allowing them to discover their passions.'

This was exactly what I had been trying to do for the past few years. There were a number of sports that I took on where I would bring David with me, and we would take classes together. Spartan training and Ninja Obstacle Course Racing were two such disciplines.

Dr Rafanan suggests to parents who want to encourage children to start sports, to start when the child is around five to seven years old, to enhance physical development and moldability. More and more schools are diversifying their sports programmes to develop future star athletes.

On the other hand, countries like New Zealand have a different perspective when it comes to their sports culture. Scott Larsen tells me that New Zealand's sports culture is shaped by its small population and the need to develop every child into a diamond, rather than churning out a lot of kids and letting the cream rise. The psychology of getting a child to sustain their interest and drive in sports is crucial to producing world-class athletes, and New Zealand's approach is more deliberate and focused on developing each child correctly.

In the meantime, I'm hopeful that my son will eventually find his sport. I've already taken him to his first tennis lesson, which he had asked for. I feel I've come full circle as tennis was the same sport my father had introduced me to. These days, when I take my son to his tennis lessons, I make sure to bring along my now eighty-two-year-old father Dave to hit a few balls. My father said if not for tennis, he would probably not still be alive at this point.

Ageing Strong

Movement and exercise become even more essential as one ages, especially if longevity is one of your goals. When my father Dave started shivering uncontrollably after we had come from island-hopping in the beautiful island of Sicogon, which is located in the central islands of the Philippines, we had to travel in choppy seas in the middle of the night to the main island to get him to the nearest hospital.

His pneumonia from that trip would cause him to be bedridden and lose not just muscle mass but also his motivation to move. He would eventually make frequent visits to the ER, usually for the same condition. His health and vitality deteriorated through the years, and during the pandemic, we thought that if he caught COVID, he would have a hard time recovering.

Somehow after the pandemic, he started moving again. He was able to regain his appetite, and recently, we were able to have him restart a regular gym routine at home.

I have seen firsthand the difference of geriatric exercise and its positive impact through Coach John Rainiel 'JayR' Felix, and his work with my father. Coach JayR is a licensed nurse who pursued a career in preventive medicine and the fitness industry. He has been involved in sports and fitness for over two decades and holds certifications in personal training, functional training, and rehabilitation.

The regimen Coach JayR built for my dad focuses on balance training, as maintaining balance is crucial for elderly individuals. They started with simple exercises, such as activating the toes, which are often overlooked but essential for balance—pressing down on the ground with the toes, activating different parts of the foot, and then gradually progressing to more challenging movements. Dad went from struggling to stand on one leg for a few seconds, to surpassing the recommended fifteen-second mark.

Additionally, Coach JayR focused on stability training, gradually increasing the difficulty by adjusting the parameters of the exercises. This included widening stances and adding weights to further challenge Dad's stability and strength.

Progress was carefully monitored, with Coach JayR assessing my father's balance, coordination, flexibility, and strength over time.

Initially, Dad found the routine challenging, both physically and mentally. Positive reinforcement played a significant role in his progress, with Coach JayR providing encouragement and reassurance throughout the process. I saw how Dad's confidence grew as he achieved milestones, such as walking longer distances and navigating stairs with ease.

Furthermore, strength training was incorporated into the regimen, with Dad making impressive gains in muscle strength and endurance. His ability to perform exercises with heavier weights and shorter rest intervals demonstrated significant improvement.

Beyond physical fitness, Coach JayR also emphasizes the importance of maintaining proper posture for the elderly. These involve exercises to strengthen the back and neck muscles.

From what I observed with Coach JayR's approach, exercise for the elderly should focus not only on improving physical fitness but also on enhancing one's overall well-being and quality of life. Through dedication, encouragement, and tailored exercises, my dad has made remarkable progress in just a few months. My dad just turned eighty-two this year and looks stronger now than he did five years ago. We hope he keeps this up and serves as 'fitspiration' for other seniors who feel they can no longer get into an exercise programme or routine in their advanced years.

He always credits the fact that he quit smoking two packs a day at the age of forty and started playing tennis the same year, which turned his health around. He would eventually play the sport for the next twenty-seven years or so, before giving it up entirely as he felt it was too physically intense for his age. These days, with newfound strength and confidence in his movement, he has been open to the idea of hitting balls again, and I make sure to always invite him when my son takes his lessons. He may miss a few due to poor eyesight, but it's heartwarming to see him hit again, and see his face beam with happiness from doing so.

The more physical activities he engages in, the better it is for his overall health and well-being.

Mixing Things Up for Longevity

The downside of specialization or doing just one sport is that your body will always respond only to the movement and exercise that you subject your body to. Most professional cyclists have disproportionately well-developed legs compared to their upper bodies. World class sprinters have trained their bodies for speed and have very little endurance, while endurance athletes have trained for endurance and with a few exceptions, are not meant for sprinting. In some cases, muscle imbalances from overly specific training result in injuries.

I surmised that unless my life and finances are totally dependent on the outcome, it will always be good practice to mix up my movements so I can have a longer 'career' as a master athlete. I may lose out on the benefits of specificity in the short term, but this translates to more balance and overall freshness in my approach to sports. Herein lies the art of peak performance vis-a-vis longevity.

Strength, endurance, balance, and flexibility training should always have their place in any person's movement or exercise routine, and in the context of longevity, it is these four key areas that one should focus on, as also recommended in *The Maximon Compendium*.[69] Below, we discuss the benefits of each and examples of activities you can engage in, and what I personally do to balance out my workout and training routine.

Equip Yourself with the Right Tools

Home gym

Most gyms will have most of the equipment you will need to get in shape. From cardio equipment to free weights to machines. If you are not inclined or prefer to work out from the comforts of home, a home gym can, if properly set up, provide you with as much variety as any gym. Building our home gym was a decision we made when the pandemic struck, and it's been such a convenient and important part of our home ever since.

Table 3.1: Different types of training

Type of training	Good for	Benefits	Activities	My training Protocol
Endurance	Lungs, heart, overall cardiovascular health	Boosts cellular metabolism; prevents heart disease; helps with fat and cholesterol management; builds mental and physical stamina; helps with overall lifestyle improvements, physically and mentally.	High-intensity interval training (HIIT), running, jogging, cycling, boxing, jump rope/ skipping, swimming, dancing	Alternating running, cycling, and swimming within the week.
Strength/ Resistance	Bone density, muscle mass, mitigating fall risk	Builds muscle mass and reduces risk of developing osteoporosis.	Free weight exercises using dumbbells, barbells, kettlebells, or medicine balls; weight machine exercises; resistance band exercises; bodyweight exercises that create resistance against gravity; plyometrics	Strength/ resistance training at least three times per week.

Balance	Body awareness, reaction time, coordination of muscle groups, joint stability	Helps to prevent detrimental falls; muscle control and movement (balance stabilization); mobility (balance strength); dynamic control, i.e. how you land when hopping on one leg (balance power).	Bodyweight exercises such as single-leg lifts, alternating knee lifts; weighted exercises such as single-leg deadlifts or single-leg lifts on a balance ball; Pilates; yoga; cycling on a non-stationary bike	Incorporated into my strength and resistance training.
Flexibility	Mobility and independence, muscle lengthening, decreasing of risk of joint pain, strains, and muscle damage	Helps reduce the risk of injury, maintain good balance, and improve your range of motion.	Stretching; Pilates; yoga; pairing breath with movement	Always do dynamic stretches before working out, and static stretches post workout.

These to me are the most basic and practical equipment you will need to set up your home gym:

- **Adjustable dumbbells:** Allow for a wide range of weight options in a compact space, enabling various strength training exercises for different muscle groups.
- **Barbell and weight plates:** Ideal for compound lifts such as squats, deadlifts, bench presses, and rows, offering progressive resistance for strength gains.
- **Adjustable bench:** Enables incline, decline, and flat bench pressing, as well as seated exercises like shoulder presses and curls.
- **Pull-up bar:** Allows for pull-ups, chin-ups, hanging leg raises, and other upper body and core strengthening exercises.
- **Kettlebells:** Versatile for strength and cardiovascular training, offering dynamic movements such as swings, Turkish get-ups, and goblet squats.
- **Resistance bands:** Provide variable resistance for strength training, mobility work, and stretching, with minimal space requirements.
- **Suspension trainer (e.g. TRX):** Allows for bodyweight exercises targeting multiple muscle groups and offering scalable resistance levels.
- **Medicine ball:** Useful for dynamic strength and power exercises, as well as core stability training and partner drills.
- **Plyo box:** Enables plyometric exercises for explosive power, agility, and lower body strength, with adjustable heights for progression.
- **Yoga mat:** Provides a cushioned surface for floor exercises, stretching, yoga, and Pilates routines.
- **Foam roller and mobility tools:** Assist with self-myofascial release, flexibility, and recovery, aiding in muscle relaxation and reducing soreness.

- **Power rack or squat rack:** Provides a sturdy framework for safely performing squats, bench presses, pull-ups, and other strength exercises, with adjustable safety bars for added security.
- **Rowing machine:** Offers a low-impact, full-body cardiovascular workout that also engages muscles in the arms, legs, and core.

Biomechanical Foot Analysis

As a runner, it's imperative that you know your foot type and how you run to be able to find the right shoe for you. One of the more important diagnostic tests I knew I had to take was a gait analysis, courtesy of running specialty store Runnr in Manila. Runnr's founder Toby Claudio walked me through the process of analysing both my feet and gait. In the 3D Volumental Foot Scanner scan of my feet, I was surprised that my left foot was a little larger than my right at 9.9 and 9.7 in sizing, respectively. The 3D scan also revealed that I have wide feet and a low arch. From this test alone, Toby and his team were able to recommend that I needed special support or stability shoes to protect my arch.

According to Toby, people don't usually consider the width of their feet when buying shoes, which then affects comfort and performance.

In the next test, I was asked to run barefoot on a treadmill with a high-speed camera taking footage of my gait. A close-up analysis showed that my ankles actually bend inwards due to lack of arch support, with an inward ankle pronation angle of 187.7 degrees upon impact; 8 degrees more than perpendicular. This indicates that my arch flattens out upon impact, leading to inefficiency and potential knee pain. Toby pointed out that I demonstrated a strong push-off due to my experience as a runner and sprinter, but my current gait puts more pressure on the side of my feet. Upon trying out a wider shoe with medial arch support, my gait improved to

181.5 degrees, which greatly reduces risk of getting injured while running. They also recommended and fitted me out with insoles to add support for my over-pronation.

Finding Your Perfect Gym

The pandemic was instrumental in forcing a lot of people, including myself, to reconsider their usual gym memberships and just opt to just build their own at home. There comes a certain point however, where you realize that there are things that you can still do better in the gym.

Aside from the fact that there's a more complete lineup of exercise equipment, the presence of coaches and even classes give you more options. Besides, sometimes it can get really lonely and repetitive when you do the same exercises at home, which if you don't have a programme that mixes things up, can be what you will end up doing.

I discovered Kinetix Lab, a luxury boutique gym that focuses on strength training. What piqued my interest was the availability not just of a complete lineup of the best premium equipment, but coaches, physiotherapists, and recovery tools.

I feel at this point that if a gym can't offer something you can do or have at home, there won't be too much of a compelling reason for you to go if you already have a home gym.

I also felt right at home since their other top-tier gym Kinetix+, which I have access to has Technogym equipment, which is the gold standard for exercise equipment and used in the Olympics. I have the Technogym Row and Technogym Run at home, but Kinetix+ has Biostrength by Technogym, a strength machine that uses aerospace technology powered by AI to ensure maximum neuromuscular activation and proper exercise setting and execution. I was like a kid in a candy store the first time I stepped in the gym, and I knew I found what I was looking for.

The first thing they had me do was a Strength Meter + Assessment to determine my strength capabilities. The evaluation serves as a benchmark to enable the coaches to formulate a personalized fitness strategy to align with my goals. I was pleasantly surprised with how I did since I don't lift heavy weights at home, given the fact that I don't have a spotter or someone who can assist me when I lift heavy weights.

Some of my results are as follows:

Bench Press 1-rep max	: 200 lbs.
3-rep Squat	: 250 lbs.
Pull-ups to failure	: 41 reps
3-rep Hip Thrust	: 330 lbs.
12-minute run	: 2.25 km.

The Strength Meter + Assessment is meant to give coaches an idea of my strength and cardio capabilities so they can properly recommend programmes based on my objectives. It would be interesting to see how much stronger I can get as I get older if I really want to. With that being said, there's no stopping me from lifting a 260 lbs bench press again, which is what I used to lift in my twenties. I don't think I could even do thirty pull-ups in my twenties, but now I found out I can do forty-one. Age is really just a number and our bodies, if we take care of them as we age, will respond accordingly.

How would you approach your particular gym preferences? What factors would come into play? At the end of the day, whether you decide to set one up at home or enrol in your local gym, the most important points to consider would be that working out should be easy for you to do on a regular basis and should be motivating enough for it to be sustainable.

Your to-do list to achieve peak movement regimens:

- **Encourage your partner/parent/kids to join you for an early morning walk.** Introduce them early on to the benefits of feeling the morning sun on your skin and starting the day by moving.
- **Find an exercise that you enjoy and take it to the next level.** Ever had the itch to join a race/tournament? Maybe this would be a good opportunity to train yourself to achieve a sports goal, no matter what age or stage in life you're in.
- If you're already engaged in a sport that you love doing, **find a coach who is attuned to your needs** and offers you a programme that best suits your lifestyle. This applies to our kids and parents who may have different needs that specialized coaching can address.
- **Have your feet measured and assessed.** A 3D Volumental Foot Scanner and Video Gait Analysis will give you an accurate picture of your feet and gait so you can find out the kind of support you will need for your foot and foot type.

Chapter 4

The Peak Performer Mindset

'Talent hits a target no one else can hit;
Genius hits a target no one else can see.'

—*Arthur Schopenhauer*

How does one define peak mind performance? Is it similar to being able to access memories from your childhood of a movie clip you once saw of Bruce Lee which then allows you to mimic the exact same movements that give you the ability to thwart goons out to get you? This is what happens in the 2011 movie *Limitless*, where Bradley Cooper plays struggling writer Edward Morra, a man who has lost all motivation and inspiration in life. When introduced to a nootropic drug called NZT-48, he gains the ability to fully utilize his brain and allows him to drastically change his life and lifestyle.

Due to its irresistible premise, the movie gained a cult following—after all, who wouldn't want to take a pill that will allow you to increase your brain's ability to function?

In real life however, scientists have repeatedly debunked this neuromyth after researchers as early as the 1930s tried to explore various regions of the brain through electric shocks, to no avail.[70] Either way, who wouldn't want an easy way out, especially if it comes in a magic pill that can instantly change your life?

In the movie, it's interesting to note though what the character Edward Morra did first after he downed NZT. For some bizarre reason, he started cleaning his pigsty of an apartment. Perhaps we can all learn from this.

A cluttered space is a cluttered mind—it has been scientifically proven that a clean environment not only alleviates anxiety, but also helps you focus on more important tasks later on.[71] Making up your bed first thing in the morning upon waking up does not only put you in the right mindset and sets up intentionality, it likewise gives you an opportunity to clean the first space that you left from your previous day.

It is a reset, and a reset that begins with a clean space.

If your mind is in the same state as your bedroom right now, how productive and relaxed will you be?

For this chapter on the mind, I would like to invite you to begin with a clean and clear headspace. I'll be sharing some thoughts and concepts not just for peak performance per se, but for anyone who feels their world may be a bit overwhelming and just in need of a reset.

The Mind at its Peak

The mind is central in achieving peak performance. Not just in the medical sense, but in how goals are set, achieved, and assessed. In the face of challenges, unexpected events, and other external factors, how will your mind absorb and react?

In this chapter, we delve into the multiple psychological factors that influence performance outcomes, because the needs and functions of our brains are complex. When talking about peak performance and the mind, the goal is to not to increase your IQ or the greatest number of active brain cells. In this chapter, I look at how resilience, mindfulness, and the pursuit of happiness can be some of the most important attitudes to incorporate in the peak performer mindset.

Mind Resilience

Life is filled with challenges that we cannot control, whether it's unexpected circumstances, events or people, training the mind to be more resilient is one way to take care of your mental wellness. Building resilience means being able to cope with whatever life throws at you. There's a saying, 'Life is not about how many times you fall down. It's about how many times you get back up.'

The National Health Service (NHS) UK provides some strategies in building resilience,[72] starting with what you're good at, followed by thinking of difficulties you have already overcome. Focusing on your current skills will help you create a better image not just of yourself but of the situation or challenge you are currently facing. This is an example of positive psychology, which has been recently linked to health and longevity.[73] Finding this image or metaphor to help in difficult times, as well as taking some time to plan, helps in building mind resilience. Finally, it is important to reflect, recognize, and reward efforts in getting back up to fight another day.

By identifying your strengths, starting back up will be easier. Recognizing your skills and your own expertise will boost your confidence and help you realize that whatever you're going through is nothing you cannot handle.

Mind resilience might not be the first thing one would think when one meets muscle-bound pro Spartan athlete Kevin Donoghue for the first time. However, under his muscular physique and the action-packed shots people would see when they look up his name, it's not hard to realize that what he does takes a lot of inner strength and mind resilience. On a virtual call with me from his pickup truck in upstate New York, we bantered and talked about how he keeps both his body and his mind in peak form.

I've had the privilege to compete alongside Kevin back in 2022 for the World Obstacle Ninja World Cup No. 1 Obstacle Race held in Manila. He was flown in primarily to serve as the emcee for the event by the organizers. I honestly didn't know anything about him, except for the fact that he was supposed to be a legendary Spartan pro racer. Then when word got around that he was entered in the same age group that I was in, I sat up and took notice.

Kevin was battling jet lag with barely a few hours of sleep as he just flew in from the US. I myself was just two weeks recovered post-COVID competing in a sport that I had only started training for a month prior. I'm amazed by how he clearly remembered the event: 'I'd been up for I think about twenty-six hours straight at that point. And I'm like, you know what, I could give ninety seconds of the best of myself and go out and actually race.'

The two of us ended up battling for second place in the race, with him beating me by maybe a second. Placing third seemed like first to me in retrospect when I had a chance to actually look him up.

With more than 150 podium finishes in his career as a Spartan pro athlete, Kevin has developed his own bulletproof mindset and lifestyle, which was evident by how he managed to still land second after travelling halfway across the globe twelve hours prior and emceeing an entire event. Aside from not consuming any alcohol and eating healthy, Kevin shares a specific belief that keeps him going, which is being afraid of losing: 'I can tell you all the times I lost, and then I can tell you very rarely a lot of times I win because I'm more afraid of losing than I am happy with winning.'

While many pro Spartan athletes' careers only last four or five years, Kevin has been in the sport since 2015, with no reason nor need to stop anytime soon. When I asked him how he is able to keep his eyes on the prize for such a long time, he answers:

> One is going back to really loving the process, right? If you're putting in all this hard work, you want to leave something behind, and people can't talk about this sport and not mention your name in there. [. . .] Leaving a legacy to me is very important.

Along with his fear of mediocrity, Kevin also believes that it's important for the mind to be surrounded with like-minded people. High achievers never really gravitate towards or get along with mediocre people. His love for the sport doesn't just make him feel good, it makes him feel almost superhuman:

> If I'm ready to do [racing] at a high level, I'm ready for any other challenge that comes around in this world. It forces you to be an absolute, formidable force physically, mentally, spiritually, and emotionally to be able to tackle any task, any challenge at any level, and any degree of physicality anywhere in the world.

Finally, Kevin keeps it simple when it comes to advice:

> Just take one thing that you're awesome at or passionate about and give that all your effort. Go in with all your might, go in with all your passion, go in with all your strength and be great at that one thing. And you're going to go to the heights that you've never seen before.

Building mind resilience doesn't happen overnight. It's the compounding result of putting yourself in a mental state that allows you to consistently show up for yourself and for others so you can perform at your absolute best. Just like working out the physical body, it takes time, effort, and discipline to achieve a better mindset.

Adaptability Quotient

Much has been said about intelligence quotient (IQ) and emotional intelligence quotient (EQ) and their roles in success. While both are important, the current pace of change in our planet demands that we keep up and instead focus on improving our adaptability quotient, or AQ, both as individuals or as units at home or at work.

The quest towards peak performance means being able to recognize that there are external factors that we cannot control, so we must learn how to control ourselves before it controls us.

The AQ model has several dimensions,[74] with the primary abilities being grit, mental ability, mindset, resilience, and unlearn. Large organizations have been investing in AQ in improving their business models as needed, instead of sticking to rigid structures or the usual proven formulas. Author Nancy Giordano adds that, 'Wonder, diversity, humility, empathy and collaboration, flatten organizations. That, combined with a strong sense of purpose, are the kinds of practices that strengthen our adaptability quotient.'[75]

Working on Your AQ

While grit, mindset, and resilience are already common leadership or peak performer skills, mental ability and knowing unlearning remain underrated abilities to master. Here are some tips to boost your AQ levels[76]:

- Be curious. A learner's attitude makes it easier to both learn and unlearn concepts and strategies for improvement.
- Be accountable. Especially when it comes to how you spend your limited time, being self-accountable helps in staying motivated to adapt.
- Be courageous. Stepping out of your comfort zone, asking the hard questions, or initiating the first contact can be terrifying, but it's the only way to show yourself that you *can* and *will* adapt.

Stress Management

Stress is inevitable, but long-term or chronic stress can affect both the mind and the body.[77] When one experiences stressors over a prolonged period of time, it can result in a long-term drain on the body. Here are some ways you can manage your stress levels:[78]

- **Determine the stressors.** Take note of how you usually react to stressors, both physically and mentally. What is your usual train of thought, and is it helpful in alleviating the stress you are feeling?
- **Look at the bigger picture.** A lot of stressful situations are short-lived or in the moment. If the stressor will not affect you in the long run, you can approach things in a more objective way.
- **Find your ideal coping strategy.** Some healthy coping mechanisms include breathing exercises or walking.[79]

Stress is one of the things that mindfulness through yoga and meditation can address. I talk about this later on in this chapter. In an event where I got to meet the renowned Indian spiritual leader and humanitarian Gurudev Sri Ravi Shankar, he imparted something important when it comes to having a strong mind: 'A strong mind can carry along a weak body. But a weak mind cannot carry along a strong body.'

When you learn how to anticipate, deal, and cope with stress, you will be able to foster your relationships better, show your more authentic self, and ultimately have more time to achieve your goals.

The Power of Storytelling

The mind is engaged by powerful storytelling. It is evident in how we appreciate books and movies. Cognitive psychologists have seen how the human mind assembles bits and pieces of experience into a story in its attempt to understand and remember. Stories or narratives tend to be more memorable than lists or tables.[80]

In the realm of business or influencing, storytelling skill is important especially for those who want to become leaders in their chosen fields. Victor Antonio is a master storyteller, and one of my sources of inspiration as a professional speaker. At thirty-six years old, Victor walked away from a cushy $20 million sales and marketing job.[81]

As he travels the world to help sales and marketing employees improve their pitches and communication skills, Victor shares how his 'SPA method' (Story, Point, Application) serves as a structural foundation for his narratives as a motivational speaker. Starting with a personal 'story', he finds a point of common experience with his audience, followed by the actual 'points' he wanted to convey. In 'application' he connects and closes the stories in his speech, making for a talk to be talked after by the audience. He gives advice for aspiring speakers in their chosen fields: 'We live in a visual medium for our business. People want to see you on stage. They want you to move around on the stage, they want us to engage. The more you can show them, you reduce their uncertainty in hiring you.'

From corporate America to motivational and sales speaking, Victor is proof that sometimes the challenge is not climbing the ladder, it's having to cut the tree and make the ladder yourself.

The Mindfulness Movement

During a recent trip to Finland, where I was filming my documentary series *Methods to Greatness*, I sought to make the most of my time with as many activities as I could fit in my schedule. The moment I set foot in Nuuksio National Park however, it's as if everything around me slowed down. There I met Mikaela 'Miki' Vuorisalmi, a yogi who reminded me of the origins of this practice: connecting your mind and body to nature, and how it can help you find your purpose.

Mindfulness is defined by the American Psychological Association as the awareness of one's internal states and surroundings, which can help avoid destructive or automatic habits and responses by learning to observe one's thoughts, emotions, and other present-moment experiences without judging or reacting to them.[82] Sub-categories such as mindful eating (which we discussed in the previous chapter) and mindful walking have also sprung from this, showing the rise in interest in mental activities and practices.

'Do you see those trees over there?' Miki pointed to what looked like two century-old trees along our snow-covered forest trail. 'I talk to them all the time.' When I asked her how she manages to do this, she explained that it wasn't so much that she started the conversation, but consisted more of listening until they actually speak to you. I honestly thought the whole thing was a bit woo woo but I reserved my judgment and tried to keep an open mind.

When we found the chance to talk later, Miki reminded me that many have forgotten how to connect to nature, as we are more focused on external factors: 'We need to listen to our heart and gut feelings which connect us to the earth.' From her home in the middle of the forest, Miki emphasized how we need to pause once in a while and revel in nature where we came from. Even those who were hesitant to do yoga find benefit from just being in nature.

Miki hopes that people will wake up and realize that Earth is all around them, and you do not have to go to the Himalayas or find the perfect guru to heal you:

> I don't think you need to run away from where you live. You just need to wake up to understand that you are part of the world, even though you live in the most polluted city in the world. But still when you open up the window: you can concentrate on the pollution, but if you concentrate, you can still find air inside there.

Miki also finds music and dancing a good way to practice mindfulness. Whether it's through a downward dog pose or to the beat of your favourite song, let your mind decide.

Mindfulness and the Body

Mindfulness is heavily influenced by the power of yoga and meditation. Yoga, specifically, is a 5,000-year-old practice rooted in Indian philosophy focused on bringing harmony between mind and body through physical postures (*asanas*), breathing techniques (*pranayama*), and meditation (*dyana*).[83] It is a delicate mixture of the art and science of healthy living practiced by millions of people around the world.[84]

Like most people I know, their initial exposure to yoga was during a group class. My initial experience with yoga during gym class was quite interesting. It was a departure from my typical strength training sessions and was a good break from the heavy lifting I would do in the gym.

Later, I would discover that yoga as an integral component of any health and wellness regimen of high performers was more commonplace than I thought. When I attended the executive programme of Singularity University in Silicon Valley, a programme for executives dedicated to the study and exploration of exponential technologies, a quick thirty-minute HIIT (high intensity interval training) session would alternate with yoga every other day.

The profiles of my fellow attendees were quite impressive. Business leaders, mostly C-Suites, entrepreneurs, and government leaders. Mostly type-A achievers. Of the 100 or so who took the one-week programme, about twenty of us were regulars in the optional 6 a.m. exercise classes. All of us were in excellent shape, and you can tell some were also former athletes. You would think that the ones who would do the HIIT workouts wouldn't be the same ones who would do yoga, but this was clearly not the case. Here, I realized that high performers need as much non-intense movement in their exercise arsenal as they do the intense ones.

This was San Francisco, and between nibbling on organic, microbiome-friendly meat alternative burgers, avocado-laced sandwiches and kombucha, the optimization vibe was apparent. Every day, our programme moderator Jeffrey Rogers would begin with a gratitude and mindfulness exercise where we were asked to close our eyes and open ourselves to our other senses and the sensations we feel. It was a great way to start what would be full days of learning and interaction with our professors and peers.

Faith and Spirituality

A lot of people think that spirituality means you have to follow a specific doctrine or system of belief. Spirituality is actually a broad concept that includes a sense of connection to something bigger than ourselves, such as nature or a higher being. Some choose art or advocacy. Whatever it may be, it's also a part of how we think, and can evolve throughout our lives.

Take Kevin Donoghue for example, who finds inspiration in Jesus Christ:

> I'll get up in the morning, I'll pray, and I'll think about what Jesus went through. And I'm like, if that guy could do that voluntarily, go through that amount of suffering, agony, the savage beating that that man took, and then [still] forgave the people around him for doing it, how could I complain about me voluntarily doing something that's fun?

Before each race, Kevin prays to be able to embrace the suffering, to embrace it as a gift: 'There's people out there suffering every day that have no choice in the matter. And I get to choose the amount of suffering I have. So that's a tremendous gift in itself. So, I show gratitude for that.' He adds, 'And I'm not shy about it. I'll kneel down right at the start line before a race. And I'm not trying to proselytize or trying to make a show for everybody else. I just refuse to be embarrassed about my faith.'

For my *Methods to Greatness* podcast, I talked to Nameeta Dargani, the founding member and president of Art of Living Foundation, Philippines. Her experience with yoga, under Gurudev Ravishankar, has not only helped alleviate physical pain, but also helped her find her own safe space. She tells me:

When I learned the techniques, Sky Meditation in particular, the Sudarshan Kriya Yoga technique, I was able to finally break out of that cycle of stress and the muscle spasms. What would happen is when I would get stressed, my muscles would go into spasm and that was obviously very painful and that sets off an emotional reaction.

Guided meditations are perfect for yoga beginners. The Foundation, however, emphasizes that following the instructions should not be given too much effort, and not to try to get rid of thoughts, as thoughts are part of meditation.[85]

When I finally got to meet Gurudev Ravishankar in person, just being in his presence was calming on its own. As a yoga guru and spiritual leader, he envisions a world free of stress and violence that he endeavours to achieve through his peace and humanitarian work, which includes visiting countries in conflict to talk to its leaders. I specifically asked him about the way we react to conflict or to other people, and that perhaps it's because there's something within us that needs to be healed. Gurudev agreed and emphasized how stress changes the way we react:

> The day you are stressed, you don't exhibit your compassion, your kindness, though you may be very kind. But when you are so stressed, what comes out of you is something which you don't like yourself.

During our session, he guided us through exercises and meditation that honoured our bodies, as we became more aware of our environment and eventually our minds. He reminded us of how the busy world and how our busy schedules have left us neglecting ourselves and building walls around us:

> We are all vibrations, and the challenge is how to keep our vibrations positive, in spite of all tiring moments in life, how to

keep your vibrations positive. You are feeling happy, wonderful, joyful, [but one] phone call and a derogatory remark, [it's] good enough to spoil your whole rest of the week. We have built a wall around us in our own mind, and we want to be somebody who we are not. I say, let's be natural, let's be free. The sense of freedom alone can make you blossom in love.

There is no hurry to find an answer to our individual purposes in life, and instead Gurudev suggests we adopt a holistic approach to living, balancing logic with activities like music and meditation to promote overall well-being.

Integrating practices such as yoga and meditation into daily life can enhance your overall health and sense of purpose. While it may seem daunting especially if you have little to no experience, being aware of this need to find balance is already a great first step. Embracing a mindful approach to living a more fulfilling existence begins with making that decision.

Mindfulness and manifesting

Mindfulness is defined as the 'awareness of one's internal states and surroundings'. It can help in avoiding 'destructive or automatic habits and responses by learning to observe thoughts, emotions, and other present-moment experiences without judging or reacting to them'. In psychology, therapeutic interventions sometimes use mindfulness-based cognitive behaviour therapy, mindfulness-based stress reduction, and mindfulness meditation.[86] To put it simply, it is the state being aware of the present moment. Adjacently, psychologists recommend 'grounding' for anxiety to centre someone in the safety of their own bodies when experiencing overwhelming feelings.[87]

Manifesting, on the other hand, is the practice of the conscious creation of the circumstances and outcomes that make for a fulfilling life. There is a science behind manifestation: the concept of growth mindset, as introduced by motivation and mindset expert

Dr Carol Dweck shows that believing in yourself as you aim to achieve something helps in actually writing said goals.[88]

I find this to be a true and powerful tool that has allowed me to manifest major events in my life. From becoming an entrepreneur, writing a best-selling book, all the way to winning races.

When talking to Kevin Donoghue about his mindset before any competition, he shares how he's visualizing winning and being on the top podium, using it to improve himself and eventually, actually win:

> When you get into a race—you're winning that race weeks, months, days before you get in there. That starts with you making that commitment in the morning, every time you get up to do something, that little something to make yourself better, to understand that the ability to go out and win a race and have that 1 per cent better than somebody else comes into the training and knowing that when you go in, you're willing to do that one little extra thing others won't do. Sometimes it works. Sometimes it translates into the result. Sometimes it doesn't. It's having that hope.

We are inside our brain all the time. Learning how to use techniques such as mindfulness, grounding, and manifestation can help organize daily thoughts in order to not just be more organized but have a deeper sense of fulfilment when you do get to achieve your goals. The idea of manifesting is also part of building mind resilience as discussed earlier; when you envision your inspiration or goals, you help make it 'more real' for your brain and thus easier to achieve. Call it manifestation or visualization, the important thing to take away from this is that a peak performer begins with a peak performer mindset.

Mindfulness through gratitude

Mindfulness can be practiced through other ways, specifically through gratitude. Through gratitude, one acknowledges what they have, including privileges and achievements. This level of awareness helps you foster a deeper connection with yourself.

Gratitude is the centre of Erwin Valencia's entire belief system. Erwin is known in sports circles as the former physical therapist and wellness lead for the New York Knicks.[89] What do gratitude and mind health have to do with being able to play at the highest level in basketball? According to Erwin, the connection is immense. When doing sessions with his athletes, he focuses on mental and emotional support, in addition to physical rehab.

In his graduate studies, Erwin explored the science behind the effects of gratitude in one's life, specifically when one does daily gratitude practices.

Erwin shares a story about legendary basketball coach and NBA Zen Master Phil Jackson, comparing their relationship to that of Yoda and Luke Skywalker:

> I remember once—we had an appointment to meet for treatment and exercises. He just left a voicemail, and he was like, "Hello Erwin. It's Phil. Jackson. I wanna let you know that we can begin tomorrow—it's Friday. But is it Friday? I think it's Friday, but you know what I mean. We can begin tomorrow." The reason why that was so valuable to me, and I wish I kept that recording was because of the fact that it made me realize that he was a human being after all. That you know, sometimes he just didn't know what day it was. [. . .] When you find his little quirks or notice it, then you realize he was actually human, and he wasn't just an action figure or Yoda.

Knowing the legendary coach—both as a mentor and as a friend—was a dream come true for Erwin.

Erwin emphasizes the importance of mindfulness and wellness in addition to strength conditioning for elite athletes.

Gratitude Exercise

Step #1 Do it first thing in the morning

The moment you wake up, even before you fully open your eyes, take a moment to lay in bed, put your hands over your heart and take a nice deep breath. Do it several times if you must.

Step #2 Be thankful for that breath

Some people don't get the chance to wake up the next day. The fact that you are able to breathe is a blessing in itself. Acknowledge its importance in simple words, such as, 'I am thankful I have one more day to create an impact on this world', or something similar.

Step #3 Open your eyes

From here, you can get up and start your day. Taking the time to acknowledge the blessing of life and doing it every day creates routine for the mind, which helps you focus and start on working the impact (however big or small you may think it is) that you just thought of.

Another exercise that Erwin recommends is writing down three things you are grateful for and why. You can do this at the end of the day to nicely cap off the last twelve to eighteen hours. Another example of how he practices gratitude is by savouring food and giving thanks to the hands that created it, allowing him to fully love life.

His way of living and practice has put him in the top 1 per cent of the happiest people in the world, which he had found out while studying positive psychology, through the PERMA Theory of Well-Being: Positive Emotion, Engagement, Relationships, Meaning, and Accomplishments.[90] These are the building blocks that enable flourishing for communities and individuals, based on individual factors. Learning more about these factors can help people make more informed choices to live a more fulfilling life that is aligned with their values and interests.[91]

I had a chance to invite Erwin to my home, where our goal was to prepare me for my upcoming competition. It was a great opportunity to work with someone who has such an immense wealth of experience training some of the best athletes in the world. It was a day where he had me undergo multiple protocols—from balance and movement exercises to pool training, and a sauna and cold plunge session. But what was perhaps the most impactful was the meditation exercise that we underwent before starting everything.

Erwin had me take a comfortable position in the living room, and initially had me inhale essential oils to prepare myself for what we were about to do. He then invited me to do a gratitude exercise.

One-on-one gratitude exercise with Erwin

Erwin: Are you ready to rock and roll? Let's do it. Here you go. Three deep breaths in. Breathe in through your nose, breathe out through your mouth.

Slowly continue to close your eyes and settle your hands on your lap.

Find yourself a comfortable position, making sure that you feel grounded in this current space. Begin to feel the heaviness of your feet on the floor, your hands in your lap, and your back on the chair. Notice your belly rising and falling with every breath for the normal rhythm of your breath.

Welcome to the now. Remember everything prior to this moment is not only in the mind, today's mantra is awareness. As we go through today's practice, allow yourself to be aware of your surroundings. As well as allowing yourself to also be aware of what's within. Allow your breath to be your guide throughout this practice, giving you the opportunity to rise and fall within and to rise and fall outside. Now, as you continue to get yourself settled in your seat with your breath as your guide, begin to open your senses to this current moment. Slowly hear the sound surrounding you. The AC. The faint sound of a game being played upstairs. And the faint sound of the dog that's outside. Allow yourself to listen to everything that's around you. And let us pass accordingly. Noticing that sound, but not necessarily holding on to it.

And now, use your sense of feeling. Feel the space around you. Notice the texture of your jeans underneath your hands. The softness of the carpet beneath your feet. The bounciness of the pillows that you're sitting on. Notice this at this present moment. Once again, not holding on to it. And now, use the sense of taste and smell reminding yourself the scent of the peppermint that you just smelled. Tasting whatever it is that you had for lunch and remembering that present moment.

Now, let's go back to your breath. Allow yourself to breathe in the normal way. The normal rhythm and the normal cadence. Breathing in through your nose, breathing out through your nose, slowing that down, allowing your belly to rise and fall with each breath.

And now, let's think about one person that you're grateful for. See that person in front of you in your mind's eye. The joy that person brought, the memories and the moments that you shared with that person. If that person is in front of you as you see them say thank you for allowing you to have that moment with them right now. If that person in that moment brings a smile on your face, allow that smile to populate.

And now, allow yourself to go back to the breath. Your breath is your anchor. Notice the belly rising and falling with each breath. Breathing in through your nose breathing out through your nose. Remind yourself that you are here and now in your beautiful home.

Know that you can use your breath at any given point of time; when you feel stressed, when you feel angry, or even when you feel joy. Because it brings you back to this place. And now, with a sense of awareness and the overall feeling of gratitude knowing that you can come back to this space, slowly allow yourself to come to this present moment. Begin to wiggle your toes slightly, move your fingers slowly and gently roll your shoulders back and whenever you're ready and when you feel called to, slowly open your eyes and rise.

Take your time get into that breath and remember where you are.

John: When you asked me to think of someone, I automatically thought of my wife Monica. I always say I love you to her on a daily basis, but I think I don't communicate enough to her how much she really means to me and how thankful I am for having her in my life. I mean, we've been married for over nine years, celebrating our tenth anniversary next year. But I think to this day I still lack the ability to totally surrender everything to her.

She's been with me through everything. I'm really grateful for her. And yeah, I think I just really need to tell her more how much she means to me.

Erwin: What stops you from sharing that with her, such a simple gesture?

John: I mean, like I said, I do say I love you all the time, but . . . sorry (I start to tear up).

Erwin: There's no sorry. We're just living in this present moment. And in this moment, what you feel and what you felt was to share a feeling of how much you love somebody. And knowing that there's something that you continue to do more. So, there's no sorry. It's just awareness. Thank you. And now the question you have to ask yourself is, what do you do next?

John: I thought this (session) was supposed to be for a sports performance (laughter).

Erwin: Well, part of sports performance is allowing yourself to understand where you are at this current moment, the present. And if your current truth is being able to find ways to be a better husband, then this is the truth that you're in at this moment. Because in order for you to perform at the level that you want to perform, you need to be all in in every possible way. You're right. That is the path to greatness, my friend.

John: It's not as simple as I originally thought it to be. That's one thing I think I'm discovering. It never is. Thank you for this.

Erwin: My pleasure. Give me a hug. Thank you for sharing that.

John: Thank you.

I must admit it was quite unexpected how the gratitude exercise turned out. What I was expecting was for the day to be a deep dive into performance and optimization, but it led me instead to the place where I needed to be at the moment. Sometimes, we get so caught up in things that we need to do, accomplish, and face that we overlook things that at our core should be the most important part of our lives that we should address, or be thankful for.

Erwin's question of 'What do you do next?' in this context is one that cannot be answered with just one act or thought or fleeting emotion. It's the process of embracing my vulnerabilities and also surrendering to them at the same time. And I know the person who is in the best position to help me accept this, and who I can learn so much from if only I let her, is none other than Monica herself.

I wanted to share the gratitude exercise I had with Erwin because I wanted you to also be able to have an idea of how to take yourself to a place where you need to be. I was blessed that day to have Erwin guide me, but I believe anyone can go through this exercise on their own. The most important part of this is to be open to your thoughts and to feelings that you may be keeping deep inside. And most importantly, if you start from a place of gratitude, the universe opens up more possibilities for you. I truly believe that, and I am grateful to have had this opportunity to also share this experience with you.

Gratitude is an overlooked concept when it comes to mental health. Embracing and expressing gratitude leads to personal growth and better relationships. Together with mindfulness, integrating these practices into one's daily life can enhance overall performance and more importantly, well-being.

Mindfulness with age

If we are lucky, we will get to experience the cycle and circle of life to its fullest and grow old in this world. My wellness and peak performance journey has brought me to Switzerland, a country with one of the highest life expectancy rates in the world.

My itinerary included a stop in University of Zurich, where I was able to have a very long and insightful conversation with esteemed lifespan developmental psychologist Dr Burcu Demiray from the Department of Psychology. Her research examines cognitive activities in everyday life across different age groups, focusing on ageing and psychological well-being.

One of the goals of her study is to change perspectives on ageing, or healthy ageing, as I have learned in my conversation with Dr Demiray:

> I think many people are scared of ageing. And they would like to reverse it, right? And there's a lot of initiatives about anti-ageing or longevity work that focus on medical perspectives that try to prolong lifespan. But again, what we are trying to do is show that older adults can have meaningful and very happy lives, even in very, very old ages with the presence of diseases.

There is a lot of ageism and myths surrounding ageing and cognitive abilities. When it comes to mindfulness, she says:

> Mindfulness, I believe, is trying to stay in the moment being aware of the current circumstances, the current stimuli around us being perfectly aware, but non-judgmental of what's happening around us. And this feeling of acceptance, or what's happening in the moment.

She shares some of the practical mindfulness exercises that she's learned throughout the years:

- **Socialize**
  'Go touch some grass' has never been more relevant. Going outside and socializing with neighbours, community members, even animals, can prevent further cognitive decline. From small talk to meaningful conversations, humans are naturally social creatures.

- **Reminisce**

  One of the activities Dr Demiray has observed in late life is the act of reminiscing:

  > Although it is a natural common activity in every stage of life, it's especially emphasized in older age, because they have this huge life story behind them. And there's a lot to reminisce about and to make meaning of.

- **Listen**

  When talking or reminiscing with someone about the good old days, it is also important to listen:

  > Be curious, and maybe enrich that experience by asking questions that will lead to additional memories to discover. Because research shows that reminiscence has some positive functions, and that those can really lead to higher psychological wellbeing in older adults.

Whatever age group you belong in, socialization remains at the top of the ways to improve cognitive function.

As of 2022, the average life expectancy globally is 71.7 years.[92] This is a huge leap from the average of 46.5 years in 1950. Throughout the years, there are a few who beat those odds and even reach 100 years old or older, called centenarians. Okinawa in Japan was famously known as one of the world's Blue Zones, where there's an extraordinarily abundant number of centenarians. This is apparently no longer the case, as Okinawa actually now has one of the highest obesity rates in Japan.[93] Japan, overall, does still possess one of the highest life expectancy rates, and a good number of centenarians across Japan. I had the chance to have a chat with one of them through one of my best buddies Andrew, who lives in Fukuoka with his Japanese wife Sayaka.

Sayaka's grandfather Azuma, born in 1925, will turn 100 next year. His wife passed away at ninety years old and his siblings all passed at a younger age than him.

Much like Patrizia Usala and her family in Sardinia, who I discussed in the previous chapters, family and community play a key role in Azuma's longevity and sharp mind, even at ninety-nine. While he lives independently, Azuma's children visit him weekly. When his wife died, he was able to cope well, believing she had lived long and well enough. He remains very active in his community and stays mentally sharp as he continues calligraphy teaching and piano lessons, both of which let him socialize regularly with other people.

Sayaka, who graciously translated for us, believes that part of the reason Azuma has lived this long is because he is open-minded and keeps on making new friends: 'He said his life is important since it's given by his parents. So, he wants to make sure that [he] can accomplish his life [until the end]. And although his friends all passed away, he makes new friends who are younger, and he is also involved [in the] community.' Andrew also shares that all over Japan, older people still tend to move around all the time, keeping active even if they don't have an exact exercise regimen.

Azuma hopes to live for five more years. In the meantime, he looks forward to staying active in the community, as I'm sure they look forward to him being part of it.

Having spent a few days with Andrew and Sayaka in their home in Fukuoka, I could see all the ingredients present to potentially make for a long lifetime for themselves as well. Both Andrew and Sayaka ride their bikes to work. They have access to good, nutritious food and a clean and safe environment. What I will never forget however, was the time when Andrew pointed out this old man to me who was walking along the streets of Fukuoka. 'Do you see that old man over there?' Andrew asked. 'Over here, it's highly likely that a man that old still has a father he is taking care of.' That made quite an impression on me, which only cemented my resolve to give my father not just the physical but also the emotional support as he enters his advanced years.

Mindfulness and social connections are vital for ageing well, both physically and mentally. By staying actively involved in the community, individuals can enjoy a fulfilling life at any age. This highlights that the quality of life in old age is significantly enhanced by social interactions, active participation, and a mindful lifestyle.

Psychology and Psychotherapy

There are times in our lives, regardless of our life stage, when we don't really feel all that good about life, our relationships, even ourselves. At the end of the day, being our best selves is as simple as feeling safe and secure in our own skin, environment, and relationships.

We cannot discount mental illnesses in this conversation. One in every eight people in the world suffer from a mental disorder[94] with anxiety and anxiety disorders as the most prevalent. Major depression is one of the most common mental disorders in the US and is a leading cause of disability for middle-aged adults. It is important to note that the prevalence of depressive episodes is higher among females, both adolescents and adults, than among males.

When it comes to peak performance and being at the top, there might be no better person to talk to than Miss Universe herself. Famously known in the Philippines for trying out for the local crown twice before making it in her third try, Pia Wurtzbach brought home the crown in 2015 after another famously known blunder by host Steve Harvey during the announcement of winners. Pia, as you may guess, was not announced as the winner, and it took Steve Harvey a while for him to correct himself and announce that Pia was indeed the winner of the crown.

But heavy is the head that bears the crown, as underneath the glamor and cheers, Pia suffered through numerous mental health issues such as childhood trauma and eating disorders. Now, through her platform and as a UNAIDS Goodwill Ambassador for Asia and the Pacific, Pia aims to remove the taboo from talking about mental health, as well as speaking out against cyberbullying and supporting people living with HIV as well as the lesbian, gay, bisexual and transgender (LGBT) community.[95]

Pia was at first hesitant to seek psychological help. But after a few sessions with a psychiatrist both in New York and Manila, she realized how helpful it was for her, as she shared with me in my *Methods to Greatness* podcast:

> I thought to myself, why did I never do this before? Like I had to wait until I was twenty-six years old to talk about my childhood trauma, to talk about my life, to talk about my struggles. And I already won Miss Universe. So why is this manifesting itself now at a time where I should be living my life? Cause I just got my big dream. But [. . .] you know, fame or money doesn't buy happiness—whatever issues that you are bearing inside that you are not dealing with, you're not facing, will come back and will haunt you again in your adult life.

After her stint as Miss Universe, Pia is now focused on her business and advocacy work, specifically helping other beauty queens through their own platform: to empower women beyond just pageants, covering real-life topics like relationships, family, and body image issues. 'The Queens', a platform she co-runs with two other beauty queens, Bianca Guidotti-Santos and Carla Lizardo, provides free resources like workbooks and discussions to help other women.

Another peak performer I've had the privilege to work with and interview is Jose 'Jomag' Magsaysay Jr, known in the Philippines as the founder of Potato Corner, a french fries business that started with one cart in 1992 and has grown to more than a thousand franchises nationwide and several hundred overseas. Our conversation was supposed to be about his business and how he is dedicating more time to his family. But then he brought up how psychotherapy helped him, even with just a single session, more than thirty years ago.

Around this time, the idea of going to a psychiatrist was still very much taboo, especially in Asia. People were scared to be called crazy. It was also worse for men, who were deemed weak if they sought psychological help. But Jomag realized how important it was in realizing things about himself and his relationships with his family. He realized that he had his own issues that needed addressing so he could have a better relationship with his family. The benefits of this realization extended towards his job and business, as it also helped him see his shortcomings easily.

The importance of psychological help is not just identifying any mental disorders you may have or finding the right medicine to help your brain. In its simplest form—talking with someone—it can immediately help alleviate anxiety and mental burden. If you are still in doubt, remind yourself that your brain is an organ: much like your stomach or lungs, it can get sick and need help from time to time.

As a Bachelor of Science in psychology, I've always been fascinated with the way the human mind works. When it comes to my own issues, I've always assumed that I could self-process my thoughts which is, of course, wishful thinking and just plain impossible.

The first time I ever sought professional help was during the pandemic. There were a number of issues in my life that I was grappling with, and I could no longer put off the need to address them without the help of a psychotherapist.

It was a time of self-reflection and self-awareness that I had never before allowed myself the liberty to explore. I must admit the sessions were short-lived and temporary. I found, at the time, that it was a stop gap measure to fix or make sense of my current problems. The sessions were immensely helpful at the time, but I know that there are aspects of my life that need further exploration, going back to my childhood that I have yet to fully dive deep into. This is a work in progress for me, and something that I will continue to pursue in the future.

The Pursuit of Happiness

No matter what pursuit you may have in life, happiness, at the end of the day, may be the one thing that binds us all.

At the top of the UN-sponsored World Happiness Report for the seventh year in a row by 2024, is Finland. I chanced upon this fun fact, and eventually reached out to the Ambassador of Finland to the Philippines, Juha Pyykkö, to try to find out more. While he gave me a brief introduction about the country, we both agreed that it would be best for me to find out for myself. A few months later, I was travelling over 9,000 kilometres on a red-eye flight from Manila to Helsinki with my cameraman in tow. We were dead set on unravelling this mystery for my documentary series *Methods to Greatness*, and certain it would be quite the adventure.

When I first arrived in Helsinki, I sat down in a park across from our hotel and watched people passing by. One question immediately popped in my head: 'Aren't these supposed to be the happiest people in the world?' It was freezing cold, no one was smiling, and people pretty much kept to themselves. I had assumed that happiness meant constant smiles and greetings from total strangers.

I would later be educated about the Finnish cultural traits that make them who they are, and how happiness doesn't necessarily entail a montage of laughing children playing across a flower field. This is what I learned from the Professor of Happiness Markku Ojanen, over a lunch of reindeer. He shared with me the simple inner workings of happiness, the focus of his study for almost three decades.

Professor Ojanen found himself being given the title when he published a paper summarizing all the studies and related concepts to happiness, such as well-being, life satisfaction, and the meaning of life. He then continued with his work, surveying thousands of citizens in Finland and determining happiness levels with numerical rating scales.

When asked how happiness is studied, he tells me: 'The answer is very simple. You have to ask people. And you have the scale from zero to ten. Of course, ten means that you are very, very happy, very satisfied, and zero that you are not happy any more.'

It amazed him how people he's asked don't take too much time to answer, and how the answers came naturally. 'There are not so many secrets in happiness. Most of the facts are quite familiar to people,' he tells me. Through his research, he boils down happiness to several factors.

Life satisfaction

At the foundation of happiness lies life satisfaction. Specifically, how people's general environment or society treats them or makes them feel secure.

The World Happiness Report ranks Finland as the happiest country in the world. The study has six key variables: GDP per capita, social support, healthy life expectancy, freedom to make life choices, generosity, and freedom from corruption.[96] The professor has surveyed thousands of Finns over decades to study happiness levels using numerical rating scales. Throughout the years, he's mastered the Finnish happiness patterns and their relationships to factors like basic welfare systems, income equality, personal freedoms and cultural traits that promote contentment over status contests. He then tells me that while Finnish people appear reserved in public, they have high social trust and value reliable welfare systems over pursuing loftier individual status and wealth.

Basic welfare provisions

When one's basic needs are met, it is easier for them to work, learn, and live. Access to education, healthcare, income equality, and personal freedom brings about trust within communities. At the bottom of the World Happiness ranking is Afghanistan, a country rife with political, social, and economic instability. It has been in a state of war for so many years that citizens find it hard to fulfil even the most basic needs.

While Professor Ojanen expresses satisfaction in Finland's politics at the moment, which shows the level of trust constituents have with their leaders, it also shows their privilege. 'There are a lot of studies which show that these [happy] people trust more than practically any nation. So, even though we don't smile, those other people, we trust them,' he jests.

The importance of the level of trust in the national government when it comes to happiness is also in stark contrast to the state of other nations that cannot achieve full life satisfaction, no matter their individual desires and efforts to do so.

Movement and nature

Aside from his current studies, Professor Ojanen also serves on the editorial board of an exercise journal. He has written extensively on exercise benefits beyond physical health: regular physical activity, exercise and sports are found to contribute substantially to happiness and well-being. Finns are naturally predisposed to this as I've seen first-hand.

My official guide in Finland, Sara Jäntti from Helsinki Partners, also told me that the functioning infrastructure and services contribute to happiness and contentment. As we toured the Suomenlinna Sea Fortress, a residential island neighbourhood in Helsinki, Sara described the place as compact yet well-equipped, while retaining a connection to nature. The sustainable lifestyles of residents there allow better appreciation of nature for locals. Even with seasonal changes, Sara described how long summer days energize people while the arduous winter months turn their focus inward and allow for self-reflection.

My other guide Mikael Malmivaara also spoke about how people actually forage for their food in the nearby forests, which are all accessible to the citizens of Helsinki. Berries and mushrooms are found in abundance and foraging is actually a regular activity for people.

This is where personal motivation can come in when it comes to the pursuit of happiness. Finding the time to go out to nature and exercise despite limited hours or space contributes to personal mental health. The release of dopamine through exercise leads to better memory, happier mood, decreased anxiety, and improved motor performance.[97]

Relationships and staying in the present moment

Despite all of Professor Ojanen's achievements and published studies, the professor easily pinpoints his family as the thing that makes him the happiest. He fondly recalls his marriage, the birth of his two sons, and most recently, his first grandchild.

While he looks forward to publishing a couple more books about happiness, positive psychology, and even one about lying, he tells me that these things are not as important as his family. As we reached the end of our meal and waited for dessert, I asked: 'Professor, how would you define happiness?'

He answers:

> That's one of the most difficult questions, but I have my own personal definition. You are happy when you need not think that my past years were better than now. It's being content with the present, rather than longing for how good the past was or yearning for a better future. I think this is the real meaning of happiness.

Professor Ojanen makes it sound simple. And maybe it is for some.

Reflecting on my own personal happiness, I too am most happy when I'm with my family. To me there is simply no achievement or goal or material possession that can make me more fulfilled than the time I am with and activities that I get to share with family. The conversation with Professor Ojanen was a powerful reminder that often, happiness lies in life's simplest pleasures, and that people are more similar than we are different when it comes to what truly matters.

This exploration into the nature of Finnish happiness underscores a fundamental truth: happiness is not a destination marked by grand achievements. Instead, it is found in the simple, everyday moments and the connections we nurture with those around us. It's a reminder that, despite cultural differences, the essence of happiness is remarkably similar worldwide. By embracing mindfulness, staying socially engaged, and appreciating the present, we can enhance our well-being at any age and life stage.

This part of my journey towards peak performance has shown me that happiness is a universal aspiration, deeply rooted in our connections with others and our ability to live mindfully in the here and now.

Your to-do list to a peak performance mindset:

- **Daily gratitude practice.** Begin with the starter gratitude exercises from this chapter and try to practice this for one month straight. Assess and reflect on how the practice has affected your mood and daily outlook, and how you can make this a regular part of your morning ritual. This may be one of the most impactful habits you can cultivate in your life.

- **Take a yoga for beginners' class.** There are many free online yoga classes you can follow as you begin your journey in yoga. Don't be afraid to try out and find the perfect guide compatible with your needs, and maybe even find a tribe you can join and take these classes in-person.

- **Start journalling and jot down your thoughts.** Try to not use your phone or other electronic devices: good ol' pen and paper will do and will reduce distractions as you try to write down your ideas, feelings, or other things that may have been taking up space in your mind.

- **See a psychotherapist.** You do not have to need psychiatric help in order to see a psychotherapist. If you are feeling unsure or shy, there are also many online platforms that allow video consults from the comfort of your home. Discuss with them any issues burdening you and they might help alleviate worries you may not even know you had.

Chapter 5

Recovery and Injury Prevention

Let me say this outright and I'm sure most athletes who have undergone extensive physical training and conditioning will agree. If you're a high performer you will most certainly, at some point in time, get injured. The very nature of sport or exercise is the adaptation of the body to stresses that enable it to produce a stronger body.

Some athletes and coaches even think that, unless it's due to an accident, never getting injured means you've never really pushed yourself to your limits or at least close to it. The challenge is how to reduce this likelihood of injury, as it is bound to happen to any high performing athlete. Injuries are what usually end the careers of even the best of them.

I've had my fair share of sports injuries through the years, with my hamstring injury in my early twenties being one of the defining reasons why I decided to move on from pursuing a professional career in track and field. Now, more than two decades later, I find myself returning to the sport as a master athlete, with injuries and injury prevention a bigger piece of the equation and a much more critical component of success.

As the saying goes, even God rested on the seventh day. Recovery and injury prevention is critical in peak performance, whether you are a professional athlete or not. Rest is a fundamental part of the process of your body catching up with the trauma it just went through. It is not a sign of weakness and is necessary as fatigue puts stress on parts of the body unaccustomed to it, further increasing the likelihood of injury.[98]

Sports Injuries

Let's quickly define terms. The term sports injury refers to the kinds of injuries that most commonly occur during sports or exercise but are not limited to athletes.[99] Factory workers get tennis elbow, painters get shoulder injuries, and gardeners develop tendinitis, even though they may not participate in sports. Ultimately, however, 'sports injuries' refer to those that occur in active individuals. This section focuses on the most common types of sports injuries—those that affect the musculoskeletal system.

Sports injuries are divided into two broad categories, acute and chronic injuries. Acute injuries happen suddenly, such as when a person falls, receives a blow, or twists a joint, while chronic injuries usually result from overuse of one area of the body and develop gradually over time. Examples of acute injuries are sprains and dislocations, while some common chronic injuries are shin splints and stress fractures.

The Evolution of Athletic Injury Treatment

One of the most important aspects in my journey towards peak performance is my athletic capability. Going back to sprinting and competitive sports has pushed me to not just reassess my abilities, but what I was willing to do to improve myself.

My very first hamstring injury happened way back when I was in college as a 100-metre dash specialist. Sprinters are notorious for pulling their hamstrings due to the extreme forces required to drive one's body from zero to top speed in as little time as possible.

Most times, age is just a number—but the fact of the matter is when it comes to physical strength, age is a very important number to consider. While I am confident that I was able to keep myself active, it is still important that I make up for any gaps with meticulous training, recovery, and strategic planning.

When I started training again to compete at age forty-five, I had no idea how far my physical capabilities were now from my peak in my twenties. I knew I was still in shape, but competition shape was something I had not subjected my body to for years. Though I exercise most days, how would my body react to back-to-back heavy training days? How fast can I recover and how far can I push my body?

The answer came soon enough when, two months into training, I strained my left hamstring. It was all too familiar as it was the same issue I had when I retired from the sport. One thing that I was thinking in anticipation for this kind of thing happening again, is that more than two decades later, sports science and sports medicine should be able to help me in ways exponentially better than in the early 2000s.

I had approached the idea with a bit of trepidation but with a lot of hope. In my mind, my body would follow whatever I *believe* it could still do in my mid-forties. The rude awakening came when, after the grind of training was taking its toll, my hamstring injury reappeared. The memories all came rushing back. My old injury, my nemesis, my old friend, we meet again.

I began with my standard warm-up of a mile around the oval. I would then do drills and work my way to the actual workout, which would consist of sprinting five sets of 100 metres. It was on the last 100 that I felt it. Those who've strained or pulled their hamstrings before know that most times a hamstring strain comes without warning. You're totally fine as you run at top speed and the next thing you know you experience a piercing pain that forces you to a limping mess almost too painful to even watch.

I knew the pain all too well to know that I had just done something I was concerned about from the get-go. I headed home and did what I always knew to do: get my hamstrings on ice as soon as possible to address the swelling and follow the R.I.C.E. method: rest, ice, compression, elevation.

The following day I managed to get myself to a doctor to get a diagnosis. I asked around for who was the best in the field, and I was eventually introduced to Dr Edgar 'Gar' Eufemio, chairman of the Department of Orthopaedics of the Cardinal Santos Medical Center in Manila, and owner of Peak Form Sports Recovery Center.

The clinic is a combination of his practice and modern medical equipment that can address injuries of varying types.

During our first conversation, Dr Gar emphasized the most important things injured athletes should focus on: conditioning, recovery, and proper training. He also examined my left hamstring, which revealed strain potentiality, and deemed early treatment crucial for recovery.

> [Sprinting] is a very explosive event. The more explosive an event, the higher the chance that you will actually have an acute injury, while distance events or endurance events are a little bit the opposite. Acute injuries tend to be more serious when they happen. So, if it can happen to a young athlete, of course, as we get older, the risks also become greater. So having a more seasoned, or a more senior athlete engage in more explosive events always will pose a greater risk of getting an injury.

Dr Gar also addresses worries about my hamstring, which can become a source of chronic pain or injury later on. After sustaining an injury, the next step should **always** be to see a doctor.

'It's hard to fix something that you have not diagnosed properly,' he tells me. Time is of the essence when it comes to recovery, as delayed treatment can lead to a longer need to pause all training and eventually, deconditioning.

Working alongside Dr Gar is Dr Jose Bonifacio 'Jun' Rafanan, whose specialty is physical medicine and rehabilitation. Focusing on musculoskeletal rehabilitation, Dr Jun applies varying techniques at different life stages, emphasizing certain differences. For younger or beginner athletes, honing their aptitude comes first: 'Once they realize that they have the skills, it's very important that we guide them properly in terms of the progression of their activities.'

For older athletes, on the other hand, Dr Jun emphasizes the importance of preventive check-ups to minimize the risk of cardiac death syndrome. Because ageing is inevitable, Dr Jun reminds athletes that their needs will also change:

- **Nutrition prevents muscle breakdown.** By the time you hit forty, muscle breakdown outpaces muscle growth. Proper nutrition and exercise go hand in hand.
- **Regular exercise trumps intense training.** Regular movement means your muscles are being used every day. This will help you avoid injury or strain and is also better for the mind.
- **Recovery is not a competition.** Each athlete's recovery path is unique. Following Dr Gar's words—be patient and put in the proper time to allow yourself to heal.

No matter the age, it is recommended to consult a sports cardiologist for proper evaluation and assessment, especially for those with pre-existing conditions.

Know your limits, and then test them.

Youth Sports Injuries

A lot of athletes today started out early in their lives. Dr Jun emphasizes the special attention for youth sports injuries: proper guidance and supervision is a must to avoid injuries and ensure safe participation: 'The thing that we always have to watch out for in our young population is overdoing things. Exercise programmes for young athletes must be balanced to prevent muscle imbalances and injuries.'

It is also important to consider sexual maturation when working with children in sports to ensure proper matching of exercises and training. Exercise programmes for young athletes must be balanced to prevent muscle imbalances and injuries.

While kids can bounce back faster from some injuries, preventing them from happening in the first place is better than pushing them to the brink.

Modes of Recovery

Recovery is not just about passively waiting for your body to recuperate, until you can train again. According to the Gatorade Sports Science Institute (GSSI), 'recovery from training and competition is complex and typically dependent on the nature of the exercise performed and any other outside stressors.'

GSSI primarily studies the effects of nutrition on the human body before, during, and after exercise. They share more common recovery techniques for athletes such as hydrotherapy, active recovery, stretching, compression garments, and massage and suggest that these types of recovery can enhance acute performance when utilized appropriately. They note that recovery is a relatively new area of scientific research, so athletes are encouraged to experiment with various recovery techniques to identify useful individualized recovery strategies.[100] It is important to note however, that recovery is still individualized and a regimen recommended by your doctor or trainer remains the best way to recover and avoid deconditioning.

Deconditioning occurs when an individual has been training for an extended period of time and then takes a break, making it harder to perform later on. Some people think they can recover quickly and participate in events, but Dr Gar warns to be mindful of pushing through injuries during competitions, as adrenaline can mask symptoms but lead to more serious injuries later on.

This was exactly what was going through my mind when I anchored our 4x100 metres relay team in the Asian Masters Athletics Championships. I had strained my hamstrings ten days prior to the competition, and I knew that although I could still run, my hamstrings had not fully healed yet.

My race was therefore focused on making sure I run the last leg at just the right amount of effort so as to come in fast and strong, but not overexert it so as to pull my hamstrings and totally ruin our chances to even finish the race. It was all about being keenly aware of just how much effort to put in for a strong yet controlled race, and not let the emotions of the moment and adrenaline drive me to go dangerously all-out.

We ended up winning the silver medal behind Asian sprinting powerhouse Japan, who was way ahead anyway. I just needed to have the presence of mind to stave off the threat from the Bangladesh sprinter, who wound up getting the bronze.

Still, even with the right training, preparation, and safety protocols, sometimes you still get injured. When worse come to worse, Dr Gar reminds athletes:

Deconditioning takes longer than expected.

If your fear after injury is that you will be deconditioned and your body will forget how to perform, which will then take you longer to train, then don't worry: the brain remembers. Muscle memory takes longer to decline than you think.

In my case, I kept in mind this point made by Dr Gar and trusted that even though I got injured ten days before my event, my body would still have the speed and strength built up from the months and weeks leading up to my competition and be able to do well.

Complete your recovery time.

'I'm a big believer in "one step back two steps forward".' Dr Gar believes that giving yourself a more complete time to recover will make you be able to perform better later on. Let your body heal and it will thank you.

This was exactly what I did—not rushing my recovery—which if I had, may have aggravated my condition for sure.

You have come this far.

If patience isn't your strong suit, then think of all the time and energy you have already poured into your sport: months, years, and even decades for some. Are you going to risk rushing your recovery for a single moment of possible victory, only to be permanently injured later?

Maturity comes with age and having had numerous injuries through the years. You get better at being patient when you face the consequences of impatience.

Active Recovery

Active recovery (AR) can be described as, 'any low impact activity that gets your heart rate up a bit and the blood flowing to flood the muscles with nutrients and clear out metabolic waste.'[101]

These low-impact activities include the same exercises that you used to do, with just much lower intensity. While there is still a lot of study needed to be done on the impacts of AR, interventions lasting six to ten minutes have been revealed to have consistently positive effects on performance.[102]

Examples of this could be doing light drills instead of full-on sprints, and pool workouts where you simulate your sport's movements. Erwin Valencia, who took me through the gratitude exercise in the earlier chapter, was able to teach me some pool drills that I could use whenever any strain or injury would prevent me from doing my full workouts. Simulating my sprinting form while in the pool is not only a low impact workout that prevents me from going full speed, but it also gives me some resistance that helps especially at a time when recovering does not allow me to do my full strength and conditioning programme.

Changing Things Up

Injury is sometimes not the only thing athletes must recover from. Such was the case for Marestella 'Maris' Torres-Sunang, a Filipino three-time Olympian and Asian long jump legend. Maris has had one of the longest and most prolific careers in Philippine track and field. We were actually training together back in the early 2000s, and she only retired from the sport recently at forty-one years old.

What is amazing about her story is that at thirty-two years old, in the middle of training, Maris found out she was two months pregnant. She stopped all training but chose to give birth naturally for faster recovery.

A mere forty-five days after giving birth, she immediately resumed training and made it to the 2016 Rio Olympics. One of the challenges she faced during recovery was losing weight, leading her to pivot her training regimen.

She tells me how she did it: 'We added unconventional strength training, so much so that I even pushed a Land Cruiser in one of my training sessions! It was really hard. At the gym, I carried sandbags. It was like playing, but they all helped.' She also found hot yoga very helpful in getting her flexibility back post-pregnancy.

Maris ended up breaking her own personal and country records in the long jump at the 2016 Kazakhstan Open. She credits her success post-pregnancy to totally stopping training and trying new things when she got back. The rest she was able to get while carrying her child and resuming training with unconventional methods helped immensely. This was the catalyst that eventually made her stronger and better than ever before. Maris has become an inspiration for many female athletes, particularly in Asia, when it comes to continuing a sporting career after having given birth.

Listening to Your Body

If there's anything I learned from being an older competitive athlete, it's to always listen to my body. A training plan is only a plan until you put it to work, but a training plan that does not consider and adjust to how your body feels, and circumstances that can affect how you will perform (lack of sleep, dehydration, etc.), is a recipe for disaster.

Almost all of the times when I got injured, I knew deep inside that my body was not 100 per cent that day. My attitude during my younger days was to just power through my workouts. These days, ignoring my body can come with devastating repercussions.

My sprints coach Gary Cablayan put it best when he shared how sometimes, if an athlete comes up to him to say that they don't feel good that day, he's the first one who will either reduce the load or just ask them to come back the next day.

The adage, 'no pain, no gain' doesn't belong to modern-day sports anymore, but sadly there still remain some proponents of archaic ways of thinking. I will not mention the sport, but I personally know of a collegiate coach who makes their athletes train from 1–10 p.m. and refuses to allow them water breaks. When the athletes started getting injured and getting burned out from sheer exhaustion, it was not at all surprising.

I've also had my fair share of setbacks and injuries through the years, making me appreciate all the more the importance of rest and recovery. This has prompted me to set up my own recovery protocols at home.

My Home Recovery Protocols

To ensure my optimized recovery, I perform recovery protocols at home as it is the best way to ensure convenience and that they get done.

Massage

Apart from having a masseuse come to my home for a massage, I have other alternatives in the form of a massage chair and a massage gun. These are quite convenient, with the prices of these equipment already down from their original exorbitant price points. The massage gun is a bang for a buck and the best recovery tool I've found that can help relieve delayed onset muscle soreness (DOMS). A foam roller also helps before and after strength and conditioning training. It is the most affordable option but takes a little longer and more effort to use. Regardless, it is well worth to integrate into your recovery and injury prevention protocols.

Sauna

We had a small sauna built conveniently in the bathroom of our home gym. It was actually an afterthought, and built after we had already built our house a few years ago. After getting convinced of the benefits of sauna bathing, I knew that I would be able to do it more often if I actually had one installed in our home. Though we had ours customized to fit the space that was available, there are a growing number of suppliers that sell prefabricated compact saunas, and the price points are starting to come down as well.

Cold exposure

After initially doing this by putting ice in our bathtub, I decided to go the route of converting a chest freezer to a cold plunge. You read it right. A chest freezer converted to a cold plunge. More details on this are in Chapter 6.

Supplementation

Protein, creatine, magnesium, EPA-DHA, N-Acetyl-Cysteine (NAC). These are the ones recommended for my particular sport and training protocols. Do find your own in consultation with your coaches and nutritionist.

Topical recovery

Magnesium sprays and patches. You're welcome.

Compression

2xU compression tights for recovery. The tights reduce muscle soreness and increase blood flow to the muscles, reducing inflammation and expediting the healing process. This helps you recover faster post-workout. You're welcome.

Injuries are an inevitable part of the journey for athletes striving for peak performance. Whether acute or chronic, these setbacks can derail careers if not managed properly. Fortunately, athletic injury treatment in sports medicine and rehabilitation has greatly advanced over the years.

Recovery strategies vary from active recovery to innovative approaches and along with proper nutrition and supplementation, they form the foundation of a comprehensive recovery protocol. It's also important to understand the unique needs of ageing bodies for maintaining physical health and minimizing the risk of injury.

Ultimately, recovery and injury prevention are essential components of sustained athletic success and by extension, of peak performance. By prioritizing rest, employing effective recovery techniques, and heeding the body's signals, athletes can overcome setbacks and continue pushing the boundaries of their potential.

Your to-do list to ensure recovery that brings you back to peak condition

- **List down your most common physical movements and exercises.** There are bound to be imbalances that can lead to chronic injuries. Find these imbalances and make sure to do other activities/movements that can counter these imbalances to prevent injuries later on i.e. doing push-ups everyday can lead to injuries if you do not perform exercises for your back.

- **Think of the last time you got injured.** When was this and how did you recover? Do you still feel pain from this injury? What would you have changed during the recovery process? See a doctor to address any lingering issues that can lead to worse injuries later on.

- **Practice sound recovery protocols.** Your recovery is equally as important as the activity or exercise you engage in. Invest in the basics such as massage guns or foam rollers, and possibly supplementation to help you recover.

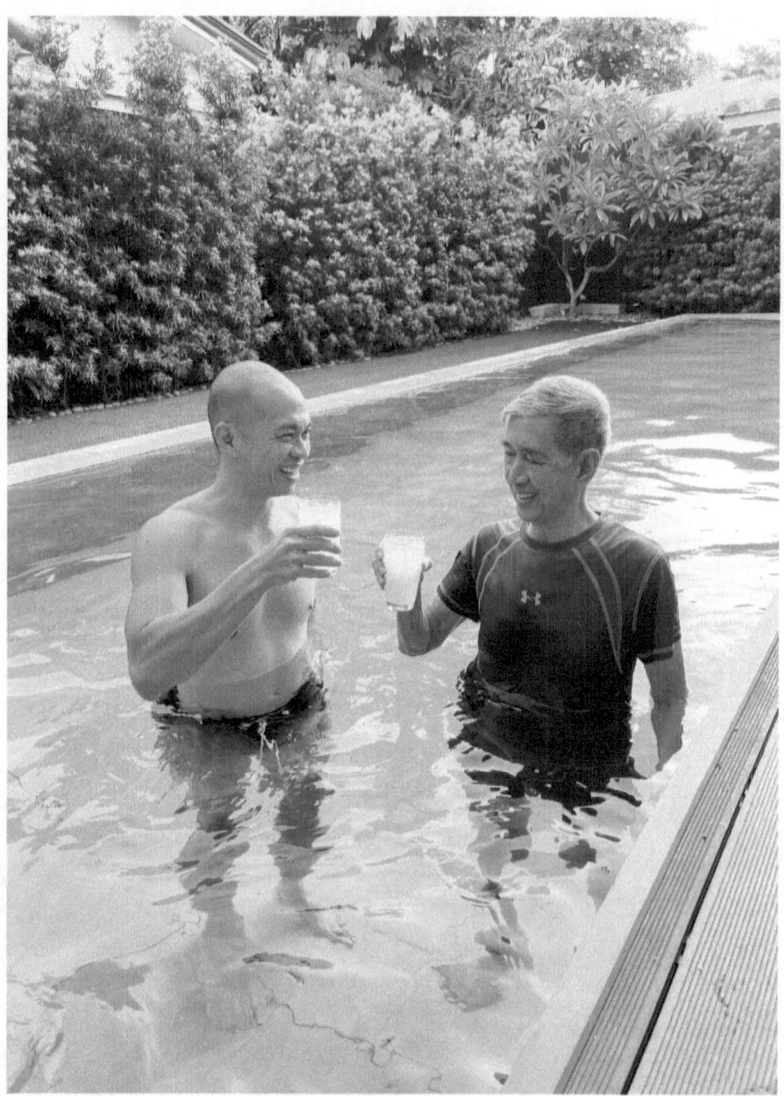

John with father Dave taking a break during a pool cardio workout

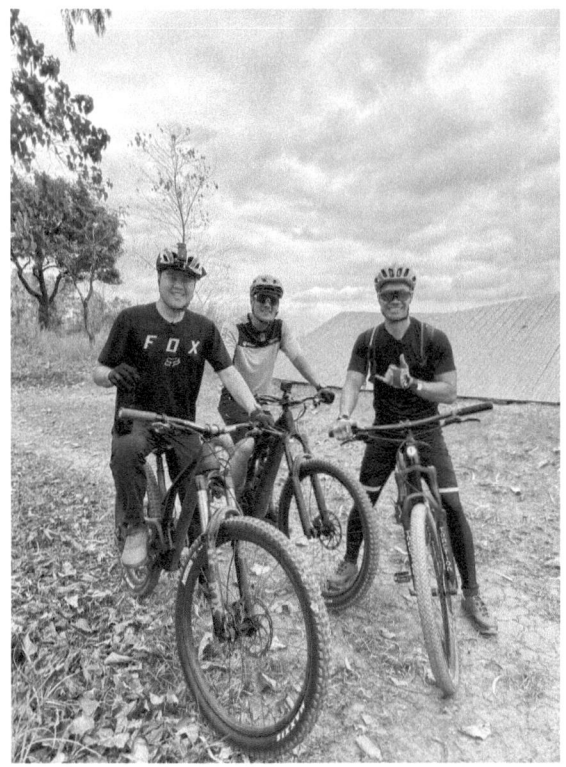

Filming on a mountain bike with Maxicare president Sean Argos and Toby's Sports president Toby Claudio

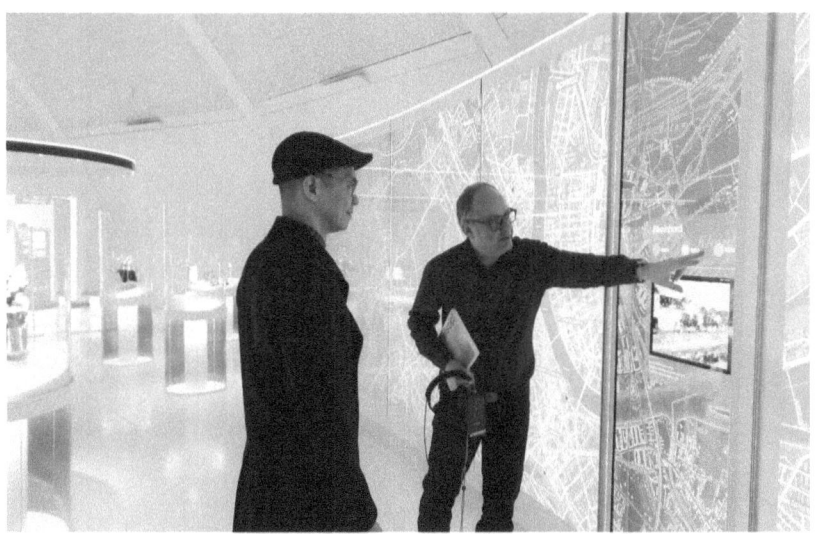

John being toured by Marcel Braun around the Novartis Pavilion in Basel

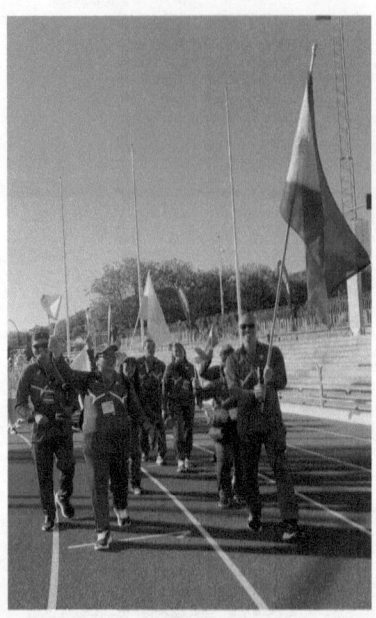

*John carries the Philippine flag at
the 2024 World Masters Athletics
Championships in Gothenburg, Sweden]*

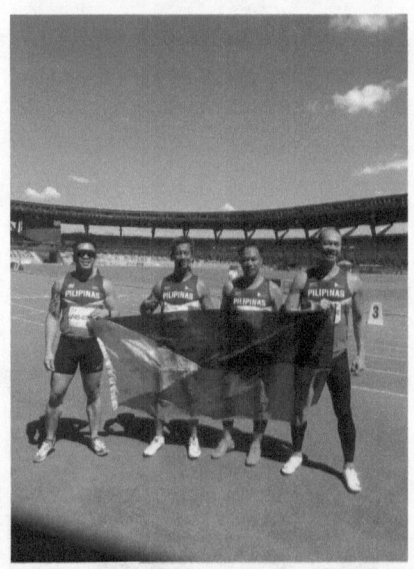

*Post-race celebration after winning the
4×100 meter relay silver at the Asian
Masters Athletics Championships*

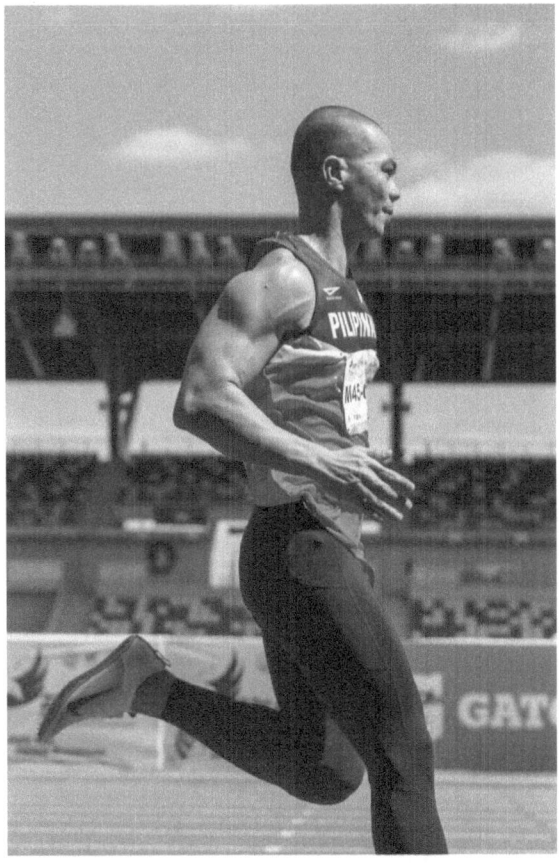

*Running the 100 metre dash at the Asian Masters
Athletics Championships*

Chapter 6

Disease Prevention and Intervention

Unlike physical injuries, many diseases are easier to avoid or manage, mostly because of all the cumulative knowledge our species has gained over many centuries. As humans, we have been cheating death through medicines and interventions and have seen tremendous success in containing and managing illnesses that would otherwise have taken down an entire village a hundred years ago. However, traditional medicine has long been focused on treating symptoms of injury, illness, or disease once they develop. Healthcare has been a misnomer for what, in most cases, is really sick care.

When my mother passed away nine months after her diagnosis, there were many what-ifs that plagued me and my family. Could it have been prevented if we had been more proactive in getting regular checkups done? Was the treatment chosen the right way to go?

My mother, who never went to the hospital in her entire life except for the three times she gave birth to us three siblings, passed away from Non-Hodgkin's Lymphoma, a type of cancer that originates in the lymphatic system. She was at stage three by the time symptoms started showing, and the tumours had already grown so big that there were very visible signs of bloating of her abdomen.

My parents' generation never really went to get their annual physical exam done, and the thinking was always to treat the symptoms. Unfortunately, in the case of my mother, it was already too late. Had we been more proactive, I believe things would have turned out different.

Losing someone gives you a renewed perspective on life. It makes you face your mortality head-on and gives you perspective on just how important health is. I want to be there for my children and our future grandchildren when the time comes.

Aside from the grief of losing one of the most important pillars in my life, the possibility of inheriting the genes that took her away from me also started settling in. When our son was born a month after my mother passed away, my wife and I were offered the option to preserve his umbilical cord blood, cord lining, and cord tissue, and store it in a private cord blood bank.[103] This process preserves possible life-saving stem cells, which he can use to combat any critical illnesses in the future. We decided to move forward with this process, since it was both safe for the baby and the mother. Moreover, we found out that it is possible for the parents, siblings, and grandparents to use the stored fluid, which has more stem cells than can be found in a bone marrow.[104] But was this a wise move on our part? Only time—and a possible future health scare or issue—will tell.

Thinking far in the future through this process is a logical step for us, as parents who want our children to have safety nets should they get sick, knowing that critical illnesses and heart diseases are the top causes of death in the world.[105] It is responsible for the death of 8.9 million people around the globe in 2019. Chronic diseases include heart disease, cancer, chronic lung disease, stroke, Alzheimer's disease, diabetes, and chronic kidney disease, costing $4.1 trillion in annual health costs. [106]

Every year, billions of dollars are dedicated to prevention and intervention for these ailments. The first half of this chapter will expound on the current best practices for prevention, intervention, and possible cures for common lifestyle as well as neurodegenerative and autoimmune diseases. The second half is dedicated to the common and less-than-common diagnostics that you can take to keep track of your health.

Lifestyle Diseases

Lifestyle diseases are defined as such because their occurrences are primarily based on your daily bad habits.[107] Here are some of the most common, including ones strongly influenced by modifiable lifestyle choices:

Prevention rather than cure

By now, you're seeing the pattern: movement and a healthy diet can and will greatly reduce the risks of getting these diseases. These illnesses even seem to go hand in hand—get one, get the other for free! So, especially for those who are a little unlucky in the genetic lottery, lifestyle modification is the only path towards a healthier body. By making healthy choices, you can reduce your likelihood of getting a chronic disease and improve your quality of life.

If you already have one or two of these diseases, we're in the same boat—but I believe the goal of achieving peak performance isn't suddenly being immune to any illness or never getting sick. It is living and performing at our best *despite* these illnesses.

Diabetes

Currently, there is no cure for diabetes, but research is being done all over the globe. [108] For Type 1 Diabetes, groundbreaking immunotherapies are being studied to see if the disease can be prevented, stopped, or even cured.[109] In the UK, the Steve Morgan Foundation has invested £50 million in the Type 1 Diabetes Grand Challenge, which brings together scientists and the community to drive forward progress in areas of prevention and cure.[110]

The same goes for Type 2 Diabetes: while there is currently no approved cure, research on weight management studies are being done, with the promise of those with the disease going into remission. This remission means that the sugar levels will be back to normal, although regular check-ups will still be needed.

Table 6.1: Causes and preventions of common lifestyle diseases

Disease	Causes	Prevention
Diabetes	Characterized by high blood sugar levels, diabetes can result from genetic factors, autoimmune reactions, or lifestyle choices.	Maintaining a healthy weight, adopting a balanced diet, and engaging in regular physical activity can help prevention. Regular monitoring of blood sugar levels is crucial for early detection and intervention.
High cholesterol	High cholesterol levels are defined as the high levels of the fatty substance cholesterol in one's bloodstream.[111] Also called lipid disorder, hyperlipoproteinemia, or hypercholesterolemia, this disease greatly increases the risk of heart diseases.	The American Heart Association specifically suggests the DASH (dietary approaches to stop hypertension) eating plan.[112] Refer to Chapter 2 of this book to find out more. Quitting smoking is one of the best ways to ensure decreasing HDL levels, paired with food intake management and regular exercise.
Hypertension	Hypertension is attributed to several risk factors, which are classified as either modifiable (diet, movement, weight), and non-modifiable (genetics, age).	Decrease risk factors and start with a healthy diet, including physical activity and high intake of fruits and vegetables. Weight management and avoiding tobacco also decrease risks.[113]

Heart disease	Leading causes aside from inborn or genetic factors are high blood pressure, high low-density lipoprotein (LDL) cholesterol, diabetes, smoking and second-hand smoke exposure, obesity, unhealthy diet, and physical inactivity.[114]	Improving heart health starts with choosing healthy habits. This also includes regular check-ups to manage other diseases you might have such as high cholesterol or diabetes.
Cancer	Caused by the transformation of normal cells into tumour cells leading to malignant tumours. These changes are the result of the interaction between a person's genetic factors and carcinogens.[115] Depending on the type and stage, numerous factors are known to increase risk of cancer, such as tobacco use, weight, and genetic mutations.[116]	Getting screening tests, vaccines for specific types of cancer such as HPV, and healthy lifestyle choices will help prevent most cancers.[117]

High cholesterol levels

While there are various medicines—usually statins—available to manage or even cure high cholesterol levels, there are also natural remedies or supplements that can be taken. Maintaining a healthy weight through exercise and good nutrition and specifically avoiding trans fats is one of the best ways to both prevent and manage high cholesterol levels.[118] Management also includes getting your levels checked as often as your doctor recommends, and more often if you have a heart disease.

Hypertension

Like the previous two, there is no permanent solution to hypertension. But once detected, hypertension can be managed, primarily by cutting salt intake to less than 6 g (0.2 oz) a day, which is about a teaspoonful, on top of eating a low-fat, balanced diet. Health professionals recommend cutting down alcohol intake, caffeine, and smoking.[119]

Hypertension is a leading cause of premature death worldwide, and preventing it begins with reducing salt, saturated fat, and trans fats consumption and instead focusing on including fruits and vegetables in your diet. Along with exercise and regular movement, these modifiable risk factors can save you from a lifetime of chronic illness.[120]

Sean Argos, president of HMO Maxicare explains lifestyle diseases like diabetes, high cholesterol, and hypertension are driving up costs and affecting younger populations. Maxicare in 2023 spent 3 billion pesos just on these three diseases, highlighting the need for preventive care.

Heart disease

Cardiovascular diseases are one of the leading causes of death in the world, caused by blockages that prevent blood flow to the heart or the brain.[121] This makes the disease one of the top priorities for pharmaceutical and healthcare companies, such as biotechnology company Roche.

In my conversation with Roche's head of Pharma International Jörg-Michael Rupp at their headquarters in Switzerland, there is progress being made when it comes to research, but there's more work to be done:

The big challenges we have as humanity in health are still [about] cancer and cardiovascular disease. That's where the excitement of R&D is, and where we as a company are hoping to have a big impact in the future. We're the biggest investor in healthcare. We spend about 16 billion US dollars every year in making those improvements for patients.

Recent technological advancements, including artificial intelligence in diagnostics and personalized medicine, also show promise in the early detection and tailored treatment of diseases. Precision medicine, leveraging genetic information, is reshaping the landscape of healthcare.

Cancer

The Big C is one of the leading causes of death in the world. Cancer treatments are classified as local or systemic: local means treating a specific tumour or organ, while systemic treatments affect the entire body. The good news according to the World Health Organization is that 30–50 per cent of all cancer cases are preventable. Major factors such as tobacco and alcohol intake, dietary factors, and occupational carcinogens and radiation should be monitored to decrease risk of getting the disease.[122]

Maxicare chairman Bobby Macasaet's prostate cancer diagnosis in 2017 was life-changing to him, in so many ways. His diagnoses began as sleep apnoea, after which more abnormal numbers in his diagnostics were found. After additional tests, he tested positive for Stage 2 prostate cancer and proceeded with treatment. He has been in remission for a number of years now:

> Ever since then, I've been cancer free. I've also been able to maintain my whole food plant-based lifestyle for the most part. And I'm really happy with the outcomes and looking forward to continuing this way for the foreseeable future.

It led him to change his entire lifestyle, with the most prominent being choosing a plant-based diet. He eliminated all animal products, including dairy, and immediately felt the changes, particularly in his weight and energy levels.

Neurodegenerative Diseases

Neurodegenerative diseases, on the other hand, are primarily defined by the loss or impairment of the neurons—the brain cells responsible for basically every bodily movement. While the exact cause of these diseases are unknown, common factors have been determined, such as age and family history.

Parkinson's Disease

WHO reports that neurodegenerative disorders such as Parkinson's Disease (PD) have doubled in the past twenty-five years. Although most people with Parkinson's first develop the disease after age sixty, about 5 per cent to 10 per cent experience onset before the age of fifty.[123] The National Institute on Aging also emphasizes:

> Some cases of Parkinson's disease appear to be hereditary, and a few cases can be traced to specific genetic variants. While genetics is thought to play a role in Parkinson's, in most cases the disease does not seem to run in families. Many researchers now believe that Parkinson's results from a combination of genetic and environmental factors, such as exposure to toxins.

There is no current cure for PD. It starts with minor to almost dismissible symptoms, such as slow movement, tremor, trouble walking, or imbalance. Non-motor symptoms on the other hand start with cognitive impairment, mental health disorders, dementia, and sleep disorders.[124]

Once diagnosed, a care plan is curated for the family of the patient. Medications and physical therapies are recommended to manage symptoms and improve quality of life. Some treatments include increasing the level of dopamine in the brain and helping control non-movement symptoms.

Psychological well-being for older adults is the part of lifespan developmental psychologist Dr Burcu Demiray's study in Zurich, where older adults prioritize positive experiences and relationships, leading to higher psychological well-being.

Alzheimer's Disease

Another neurodegenerative disorder is Alzheimer's Disease, which involves the accumulation of abnormal protein deposits in the brain. While it currently lacks a cure, medications and interventions focus on manageing symptoms and slowing disease progression. Research explores immunotherapies, precision medicine, and lifestyle interventions for potential breakthroughs.

Jörg-Michael Rupp says that Alzheimer's disease is a major challenge for humanity. The disease, along with broader cancer and cardiovascular disease challenges, is a key focus area for them.

Preventing Alzheimer's involves adopting a brain-healthy lifestyle, including regular exercise, a balanced diet, social engagement, and cognitive stimulation. Managing cardiovascular risk factors also plays a role in reducing the risk of Alzheimer's.

Dr Burcu on the other hand conducted a study among senior citizens of around sixty-five years of age, helping them start on projects that involve 'design thinking'. She notes that older adults can engage in cognitive stimulation through simple activities like brushing their teeth with their non-dominant hand or taking a different route to the gym. They should be encouraged to continue learning and staying open-minded. The project successfully launched a podcast in Switzerland—this novel project exhibits lifelong learning, where people of advanced age continue to learn based on their interests.

Older adults who feel psychologically younger have better cognitive health and longer lifespan. In our conversation, we ended up discussing how they tend to focus more on their personal past than future in everyday conversations, as well as the importance of past experiences in shaping their sense of identity and social bonding, with research showing that they tend to remember and share positive past experiences more than negative ones.

This got me thinking of my relationship with my father, who at eighty-two is still very sharp and in control of both his physical and mental faculties. My father also likes to talk about his past, about his childhood, his first career as a struggling musician, as well as business and life decisions. There is truism to the research that older adults tend to remember and share positive experiences more than negative ones. My learning from Dr Burcu is to always listen to and encourage my father to share his thoughts (no matter how repetitive they tend to be) and just allow him to share.

Autoimmune Diseases

Let me zero in on one in particular that hits close to home. Lupus is a lifetime chronic disease that causes inflammation in the skin, joints, and internal organs like the kidney and the heart. There are different kinds of lupus, such as the common systemic or cutaneous which is limited to skin inflammation.[125]

My personal experience of an autoimmune disease such as lupus is through my wife Monica, who was first diagnosed back in 2017. Her fatigued and pain-filled days pushed us to get more tests, and finally a prognosis. At its worst, her inflammation left her unable to even do a simple turn while sleeping.

But if there is a poster child for how to successfully live and navigate a life with lupus, it's her. Aside from regular exercise, and avoiding foods that can worsen her symptoms, adapting to a life with chronic disease primarily involves listening to one's body. Monica says, 'That's really my key to success: to really listen to my body and try to look at my day in advance.' This helps her ensure that she prioritizes the tasks to be done without overworking her body.

Full support and understanding from us, her husband and three kids, is important as she lives with lupus.

The Future of Treatment

Technology has allowed pharmaceutical companies to create treatments and other intervention options for many lifestyle diseases plaguing the world. Swiss pharmaceutical companies Roche and Novartis are just some of the few who are targeting specific illnesses, aligned with their companies' visions, for future populations. So far, however, there is no 'golden bullet' or magic cure-all invention from their research.

Dr Tewis Bouwmeester, senior unit head of the Department of Developmental and Molecular Pathways at Novartis, notes:

I think we always have the aspiration towards cure [for Alzheimer's]. But we also have to be very humble as to what that actually means. I think very often it's symptomatic treatment, it is really trying to understand the disease, have a bit of a reductionist approach around how disease manifests itself, and then try to translate that into a therapeutic opportunity.

'Everybody speaks about the social determinants of health and how you can address it. And the main domain evidence is always pointing towards underserved populations, ethnic minorities, or people with really specific needs,' Dr Ann Earts of the Novartis Foundation tells me. The very act of acknowledging the inequity among different countries means we are on the right path. The Foundation also aims to use AI and machine learning to identify drivers of health and health inequities in cities so local governments can use the data for policy making. She adds:

What we aim for in the Novartis foundation is healthy longevity, living in a community where you have a lot of good social contacts, where you still have a good purpose in life. This is the best condition for living long and healthy. That's well documented already. So that doesn't have to do with medicine. It has to do with the way you live your life.

Overall, disease management and prevention doesn't just enhance the quality of one individual life, it also reduces healthcare costs and promotes public health. This, in turn, helps people achieve more of their individual goals.

Proactive Health Management through Diagnostics

Disease prevention and intervention without diagnostics is like looking for something like a building block you don't know the colour of in a huge toy box. It is easier to be more proactive with your health when you know which aspect of it to prioritize.

It's also been said that married men and women live on average two years longer than their unmarried counterparts. This is attributed to many factors, among them social integration. In my case, the number of times that my wife Monica reminds me to get my annual physical exam does seem to point to the truth of that statistic.

Since I turned forty, Monica has always made it a point to remind me to get my annual physical exam done. Longevity is all about doing the right things, and prevention goes hand in hand with intimately knowing your body and its current state to better anticipate any future problems.

In this section, I've compiled the diagnostics one should undergo to be able to make sure that you keep tabs on your health. I also share and discuss the areas of concern that I have worked on and am currently working on to ensure my numbers are within the normal range as possible. I share these tests with you to give you an overview so that you can also consider them for your own health journey.

Annual physical exam

As one gets older, annual physical exams (APE) or executive checkups should be mandatory and be done as often as needed. APEs facilitate early detection and treatment of diseases, provide opportunities for preventive care, help build a strong patient-provider relationship, and contribute to overall health and well-being. In the goal towards peak performance, going through regular APEs is the bare minimum in determining one's health baseline. I did mine at our local Maxicare Primary Care Clinic, and while I was there decided to do a more comprehensive executive checkup as well to get a more complete overview of my health status.

It's important to note that not everyone needs the same sets of tests or diagnostics. For women, more specifically, certain screening tests must be done to keep track of their health. This includes getting pap smears to screen for cervical cancer from age twenty-one, a mammogram every two years when you turn fifty years old, and bone density scans for osteoporosis screening from age sixty-five or even younger.[126] For men aged fifty to seventy-five, screening tests for colorectal cancer are recommended.[127] Other screening tests such as for sexually transmitted diseases should be done depending on your lifestyle. The results of these tests are a huge part of becoming proactive in managing one's health, serving as early indicators for any underlying illness.

Blood count test and urinalysis

Starting with the blood count test and urinalysis, both of which are the most basic diagnostic tests in detecting illnesses. Complete blood count test or CBC checks the different components of the blood such as red blood cells, platelets, and haemoglobin, in order to detect infections, anaemia, or even blood cancers. A urinalysis on the other hand is the easiest way to detect any infections in the urinary tract and the kidney.

My blood count test and urinalysis results fortunately showed no specific abnormalities. However, results for my other tests led my internal medicine specialist Dr Martin Reyes into deeper discussions with me about my health.

Areas of Concern: Creatinine and Cholesterol

Creatinine

A creatinine test is taken by drawing blood and taking a urine sample. Its main function is to determine kidney health, which is exhibited by the amount of creatinine in the blood and urine. Having higher creatinine levels may be indicative of a number of factors, among them reduced kidney function, muscle mass (people with higher muscle mass tend to have higher baseline levels of creatinine due to increased muscle turnover and metabolism), hydration status, medications and supplements, or other underlying medical conditions.

Table 6.2: My creatinine test results

Renal function and normal range (for a man my age)	My results		
	2022	2023	2024
Creatinine (with eGFR) **(63.6–110.5 umol/L)**	**70**	**116.2**	**76**

Having observed my results, there was a marked increase in my creatinine in 2023. At 116 milligrams per decilitre, my creatinine levels were beyond the normal range. Dr Reyes and I attributed it to the fact that I was training heavily and taking creatine supplements during training for most of 2023.

For most people, the increase in creatinine levels associated with creatine supplementation is not a cause for concern, especially if they have normal kidney function. But it is always good to err on the side of caution, so Dr Reyes advised that I taper off creatine supplementation to bring down my creatinine levels.

I successfully brought down my creatinine to normal levels by 2024 by simply stopping my consumption of creatine supplements. As I was training again, I resumed creatine supplementation, cognizant that once my competition ends, I would be tapering off again.

Cholesterol

A lipid profile or study is used to monitor risk for cardiovascular diseases, particularly by measuring the four types of cholesterol and triglycerides in the blood. Lipid results higher than the normal range may eventually lead to buildup in the vessels and arteries.

Table 6.3: My lipid profile

Lipid studies and normal range (for a man my age)	My results		
	2022	2023	2024
Total Cholesterol (< 5.20 mmol/L)	**5.71**	**5.52**	**5.38**
HDL Cholesterol (> 1.03 mmol/L)	**1.89**	**1.20**	**1.58**
Non-HDL Cholesterol (< 3.36 mmol/L)	n/a	4.32	n/a
Triglycerides (< 1.70 mmol/L)	n/a	0.56	0.82
LDL Cholesterol (< 2.58 mmol/L)	**3.59**	**4.07**	**3.64**
VLDL Cholesterol (< 0.80 mmol/L)	0.23	0.25	0.16

My lipid results in the past three years showed fluctuations but still did not hit the ideal range, specifically in my HDL and LDL levels. While I've succeeded in lowering my total cholesterol and LDLs, my HDL (or 'bad' cholesterol) level increased between the six months from my test in late 2023 to 2024.

I expressed my hesitance to take statins, and I'm sure I'm not the first person to let my doctor know about this. However, Dr Reyes recommended medical therapy for lipid disorder as well as statin therapy due to elevated LDL and risk factors, and to just adjust medications after, if I successfully lower my levels.

Abdominal ultrasound

While not part of the usual physical checkup, I also opted to undergo an abdominal ultrasound, which uses imaging equipment to check the health of my liver, gallbladder, and kidneys. These results helped shed a better light on better ways I can take care of my liver and kidneys as I manage my high lipid and creatinine levels. My abdominal ultrasound, fortunately, showed normal results.

Stress test

As an athlete, a stress test was essential for me to find out if my heart can take on all the physical activity that I put my body through. A stress test sees how blood flows through your heart while you're exercising and can reveal problems that might arise while your heart is pumping harder and faster than it does normally.[128] Stress tests are usually done with treadmills, with EKG monitors attached to read heart activity.

Since I run all the time and push myself constantly in training, this was a good opportunity for me to see how hard I can push my heart under the supervision of a medical doctor. In my last stress test, I pushed to my absolute maximum heart rate, reaching Level 6 of the stress test after more than fifteen minutes, with leg fatigue but not chest pain or loss of breath, eventually leading me to end the stress test. My results indicate high cardiorespiratory fitness for my gender and age. This was a good sign, giving me confidence that my heart responds well to training and has good recovery.

Computed tomography (CT) scan of the cranium and whole-body magnetic resonance imaging (MRI)

While there are some red flags in my results, specifically in my creatinine and cholesterol levels, I was satisfied with how most of my results were within range, especially for a man my age. However, as someone who wants to optimize and consider all possible blocks to my health and peak performance, I wanted to go deeper.

A CT scan involves a narrow beam of x-rays aimed at the patient, producing signals that generate cross-sectional images, or 'slices'. These slices are called tomographic images and can give a clinician more detailed information than conventional x-rays.[129] An MRI, on the other hand, uses a large magnet and radio waves. Medical professionals choose which of the two are better for the patient depending on their needed scan.[130]

Through a CT scan and whole-body MRI, my doctor was able to do a deep dive into my body and its performance. These medical imaging techniques produce detailed images of organs or any part of the body in order to check for any damage, risk, or blockage without employing invasive measures.

I was glad that I received normal and unremarkable results for both.

Other Diagnostics

Aside from my executive checkup, I also decided to look upon other diagnostics. This was done in the LifeScience Center which helps patients achieve health goals through personalized health programmes guided by the Functional Medicine approach.

Group CEO Mitch Genato leads LifeScience with the goal of combining conventional medicine and functional medicine together. Conventional medicine addresses immediate health crises while functional medicine thrives on prevention and proactive care.[131]

LifeScience's approach, particularly in its potential to optimize health rather than just manage disease is one of the reasons why I took these additional diagnostics with them, as well as discuss dietary and lifestyle options that will help me in my pursuit of optimal health. Allow me to share with you in the following pages the other diagnostic tests I took:

Body composition analyser

A body composition analyser assesses the various components of a person's body composition, which includes measurements on body fat and muscle mass. These devices are used in healthcare settings, fitness centres, and research facilities to assess individuals' health status, monitor changes in body composition over time, and guide personalized nutrition and exercise plans. I've actually used the body composition analyser in all these settings, and it helps me and the teams I work with get a snapshot of my body composition. My latest results are as follows:

Table 6.4: My body composition analysis

Component	Measures	My results
Body fat percentage	Proportion of fat mass to total body weight.	10.6 per cent
Muscle mass	Amount of muscle tissue in the body.	84.2 per cent
Visceral fat level	Amount of fat stored within the abdominal cavity around organs such as the liver, pancreas, and intestines.	7 per cent
Metabolic rate	Number of calories burned at rest (resting metabolic rate) or during physical activity.	1854 kcal
Metabolic age		31

During my latest session, the Body Composition Analyser determined that I have a metabolic age of a thirty-one-year-old, fifteen years younger than my chronological age of forty-six. My results reflect perhaps a lifetime of exercise, healthy diet, and generally taking care of my body.

The most important aspect of this is not so much relying on the accuracy of the results but using it as a way to monitor changes in body composition over time. The body composition analyser is a good middle ground that balances accessibility and reliability to monitor our body composition. On one extreme would be the electronic smart weighing scales that are the most accessible but not as reliable, and on the other extreme the DEXA Scan which is highly accurate and is the gold standard for assessing body composition and comprehensive information on bone health, but more commonly used in medical and elite sports performance settings.

Whatever you use or have access to, the most important thing to know is how you will use that data to then make the necessary changes and improvements when your numbers are not ideal, or how to track the things you are doing right if the numbers are good. This way you are relying on a data driven approach and not leaving things to chance and emotions when planning your health journey.

Food sensitivity test

In 2022, I took a food sensitivity test under LifeScience to reveal specific foods causing inflammation and eventually impacting my sports performance. The specific test I took tested my sensitivity for more than 200 food groups, which examines the concentration of an antibody called immunoglobulin G (antibody IgG) in my system.

While food sensitivity is not exactly an allergy, it manifests through varied symptoms which may not necessarily be life-threatening but may still hamper productivity—like bloating, migraine, lack of energy, insomnia, etc. My results showed that I was highly sensitive to cola nuts, barley, egg white, milk (sheep, cow, and goat), pea, corn, pistachio, almond, potato, soya bean, and about twenty other things. Alternative carbohydrates recommended by LifeScience included quinoa, sweet potato, yuca (cassava), millet, buckwheat, and tapioca.

I had a borderline sensitivity to fewer (but more prominent) foods like rice, wheat, and oats. The team at LifeScience sent a comprehensive list along with a smoothie recipe guide that I could use as I made my way around these food sensitivities. The objective was to be able to have my system take a break from these foods that could be causing my digestive system to be compromised. Each of the food items I would need to avoid would be monitored over twenty-one-day cycles to ensure that the IgG[132] load is brought down to a level which leads to optimized absorption of nutrients in my gut.

What we're aiming for as well, in terms of diet intervention is the diversity of what I eat. A healthy diet is to really have a variety of foods. The more diverse the better. Whole food, not processed.

Adrenal hormonal tests

Usually overlooked unless there is a specific need or symptom, an adrenal hormone test is done to check for adrenal imbalances. Using saliva as a sample, this test 'evaluates bioactive levels of the body's important stress hormones, cortisol and DHEA. It serves as a critical tool for uncovering biochemical imbalances underlying anxiety, depression, chronic fatigue syndrome, obesity, dysglycemia, and a host of other clinical conditions that may affect our day to day lives.'[133]

A big concern particularly for men is the gradual decline in testosterone levels as a normal function of ageing. Some of the symptoms for this include reduced sex drive, erectile dysfunction, decrease in muscle mass, increased body fat, reduced bone mass, fatigue, mood changes, and others. Though I (thank God) wasn't having problems in the other departments, I was strangely experiencing fatigue in the mornings, and a general blasé feeling on some days. This made me curious to find out what my testosterone levels were like.

My results showed normal cortisol levels in all categories, but lower than average DHEA, which indicates lower testosterone levels. To address this, my doctor and I decided to go with a conservative approach and begin supplementation as well as some modifications in my diet. My nutrition plan included foods that support testosterone production, such as leafy green vegetables, garlic, ginger, nuts and seeds, beets, pomegranate, sweet potato, extra virgin olive oil, and supplementation with EPA and DHA (fish oil).

Sub-optimal testosterone levels can also be caused by not getting enough sleep, and stress. So, I made sure that sleep and reduction of stress was a priority.

DNA/genetic testing

The next diagnostic I took was a performance sensor, which analysed my athletic genes and my genetic predispositions to being either a power or endurance athlete, my maximal oxygen uptake (VO2 Max) or my genetic capability to absorb oxygen through the lungs and transport it to the appropriate muscles, my inflammatory responses and analysis of my risk of injury, my optimal performance nutrition, and a food list assessed according to my genes to help me plan my nutrition optimally.

Finally, through a genetic panel called Premium Sensor Plus, I saw how genes influence health and gave a snapshot of my physiological predisposition. This panel mapped everything from how my body breaks down and cleans out the drugs in my body to understanding my predisposition to disease conditions such as cancer (because of what my mom went through), cardiovascular health risks (including hypertension), neurological conditions, metabolic risks or how my body will age by looking into my bones, joints, eyes, and teeth health as well as my hormones as I enter 'male menopause' or andropause age.

This test is not designed to strike fear based on my disease risks but instead to empower me to understand what lifestyle factors could drive my genes to be turned 'on' or 'off' based on my epigenetics. My body is revealed to have 'good genes' especially when it comes to physical conditioning and ability to detox from chemicals and air pollutants. However, I ranked below average when it came to my oxygen uptake and VO2 max.

Mitch says:

The muscle profile you have is leaning more towards endurance, except your VO2 Max is low. Which means if you want to excel more in your endurance sports, that's where high altitude training, hyperbaric oxygen therapy, and breathing techniques come into play. [. . .] The Gene test is a reference to bump against what you're feeling and what is real to you right now. This tells us what you're designed for but how you live your life affects how that design is manifesting.

Mind map

I couldn't forget about my brain health. I was also given the Genomind Mental Health Map Diagnostics, which is designed to inform you about certain genetic associations that may influence general health and wellness. According to Genomind, the information and interpretation of the genetic results come from various sources in the public domain, which curated hundreds of the world's genome-wide association studies (GWAS) and candidate gene studies providing the framework for the test and its results.[134] This test focuses specifically on mental wellness issues, including the 7 Core Mental Health Capabilities.

Have you ever read your horoscope or had someone read your palm and tell you things about yourself? They either made sense to some degree or said the total opposite of what you believe is true. When I received my results for the Mental Health Map, I was surprised with how accurate most of them were, with a few exceptions. Though not intended to treat any disease or mental condition, the test provides insights that may be useful in understanding and improving one's general mental health and wellness, based on your genotype.

To give you an idea, the assessment below for my results summarizes the genetic findings of my genes that Mental Health Map outlines:

- **Stress and anxiety:** While I showed normal activity in my stress response, the test shows I may be predisposed to worry, lingering guilt, and nervousness. My adaptability trait predisposes me as a rule follower.

- **Mood:** My temperament was predisposed to have a Type A personality, normal outlook and mood stability, with an unflappable emotional vulnerability which makes me less influenced by social pressures.

- **Focus and memory:** My working, long-term, and focus tests all showed great results, with a specific predisposition to strategic focus, being in the zone, and impulsivity. My long-term memory trait points to improved muscle memory in my genes, which explains why I learn physical tasks quickly and more efficiently.

- **Sleep:** My circadian rhythm and ability to fall asleep showed normal predisposition, but with a predisposition to snoring and daytime lethargy.

- **Eating behaviour:** This is where it gets interesting—my tests showed that I am predisposed to emotional and picky eating, matched with a sweet tooth and the occasional fat cravings. I only agree with the sweet tooth and fat cravings.

- **Habits and substance use:** According to this category, I am predisposed to be more comfortable with taking risks, with an increased habit-forming potential. It also says that I have a tendency to drink more alcohol (which I don't) and am sensitive to the effects of marijuana (which I have not tried so I cannot verify).

- **Social behaviour:** My social behaviour predisposition showed that I am predisposed to be a lone wolf, more introverted with difficulty connecting with others. Some trust issues may also happen with an increase in wariness around others.

While definitely not required for those aiming to become peak performers in their respective fields, having knowledge on your traits based on your genetic predispositions is a good exercise to possibly shed light on why you are the way you are and guide you to make decisions driven by your understanding of your mental predispositions.

The Future of Diagnostics

Technology plays a huge part in the development of diagnostic equipment throughout the years, making it easier to detect and manage illnesses. Just like how our phones and computers have gotten smaller but more powerful, many companies have developed or are developing diagnostic machines that make it easier to access health data.

Smart watches with various fitness features are now more common than ever, promoting health and movement for everyone, not just athletes. Usual features of the latest smart devices are standing warnings, VO2 max levels, even stress detectors. In-phone health apps make it easier than ever to track movement. Apple's smart watches even have electrical heart sensors that let users take electrocardiograms anywhere. Sometime into the future, continuous glucose monitoring will be as normal as telling the time.

During my Finland trip, I was able to meet with several start-up companies focusing on creating better, more accessible diagnostics for everyone. I share some of these with you to give you a glimpse into the future.

MedicubeX Ltd

Medicube X has developed an e-Health Station™, a cubicle-sized pod where a patient can measure the most important health values in five minutes completely independently, making basic diagnostic tests easier and faster for everyone. The station measures blood pressure, oxygen saturation, 1-channel ECG, body temperature, the

AGE value that describes risk factors for cardiovascular diseases, weight and body composition.

In addition to evaluating basic vital signs, the machine enables a comprehensive assessment of the risks of cardiovascular diseases and diabetes and offers better remote receptions supported by real-time information.[135]

Myontec

Myontec specializes in 'smart clothing': a step up from the usual wrist wearables that have become common. Their products measure the muscular system directly through surface electromyography (sEMG) to let users truly know their muscle exertion and get precise data for adjustments and improvement. One example is the Mbody3 Kit Legs, which measures data from hamstrings, quadriceps, and glutes muscles.

I got to test this with Myontec's CEO Janne Pylväs and did uphill sprints in the streets of Helsinki, and later on did sprints at the Helsinki Olympic stadium, no less! The data was surprisingly nuanced as information from my leg's major muscle groups were being recorded and sent to a laptop and mobile phone in real time for every movement and stride. It gives one the ability to see and measure muscle load, performance technique, muscle balance, and the efficiency and intensity of muscle work.

Imagine having the ability to measure how your muscles are performing in real time, and if there are any imbalances or breaks in form that can lead to injuries. The possibilities for gathering diagnostic data across different sports and activities for different purposes are immense.

Northern Sports Insight and Intelligence

Northern Sports Insight and Intelligence Oy (NSII) is a Helsinki-based company that has developed a head impact tracker.[136]

The sensor measures the accumulation of forces, their frequency, and the time between impacts, which then transmits data wirelessly to a mobile app, allowing coaches and teams to monitor impacts in real-time. Imagine if coaches and athletes had real-time data on head impacts from heading footballs and getting hit repeatedly on the head in boxing matches, how would you respond to this information? And no, I did not test the head impact tracker, but I was able to hold and appreciate its unobtrusive form factor, which is small enough for you to attach to a headband or most sports helmets.

NSII aims to provide relevant data to users to make informed decisions about athlete health and safety, with a product designed to be reusable and sustainable.

I'm not going to lie—some of these tests can get quite expensive, and these new devices are definitely not cheap. In time as with all new technologies they are bound to get more affordable, and economies of scale should be able to drive costs down and make them more accessible to more patients and athletes globally.

Your to-do list to the art of prevention:

- If you haven't already, **get your annual physical exam done**, and make sure to keep your records so you can track your health and how you are making progress or declining. Prevention is the best cure!
- **Family tree of diagnosis**. Understand your own medical history by checking its roots. Determining which sides of your family are predisposed to certain diseases can help you anticipate and prepare for any genetic illness. Start out with a simple map or chart of your parents, their parents, and your siblings and cousins. Recognizing patterns, even for psychological behaviours, can give you a head start. This will also prove helpful for your children in the future.

- **Keeping medical records**. Getting checkups will be useless if you don't use them to study patterns in your own behaviour and how your body reacts to it. Keep hard copies in a secure filing cabinet, properly labelled by date. Include prescriptions as well. Make sure to keep digital copies in your phone or computer as well for easier access. Keep medical records per family member and keep track of younger family members' files so they can use it in the future. Creating this practice will also help them become more aware of their own health.

Chapter 7

Biohacking and Longevity

*'Making small changes in your environment can really ramp up
what's possible for you, perfection is not required.'*

—*Dave Asprey*

Zurich, Switzerland. After about a ten-minute bike ride from our hotel
in below zero temperatures, my cameraman Jun and I, along with
our guide Anita from Zurich tourism, were just settling into the
craziness of what I was just about to do. As we approached the
snow-filled makeshift dock, a tinge of nervousness started to creep
in. I was going to jump into the freezing-cold lake, Zürichsee.

Our documentary crew, which was composed of myself, my wife
and co-executive producer Monica, and our cameraman Jun, had
just arrived after a twenty-hour flight from Manila. Monica decided
to lay back and rest in our hotel suite. I, however, wanted to get
straight to work. Work in this case is the filming of the Switzerland
episode of our documentary series *Methods to Greatness*, a series that
traces its roots from a podcast that I started during the pandemic
which eventually morphed into a book. In the documentary, I go
on a global journey to try to find greatness in all its different forms.
In particular, finding ways by which to maximize human potential.

The impetus behind the desire to jump into the freezing cold
Lake Zurich came from a fascination with cold plunge therapy,
which had been on my mind ever since I had first heard that more

and more people were beginning to try and reap the benefits of this now ubiquitous peak performance protocol therapy. One Championship mixed martial arts heavyweight champion, Brandon Vera, was the first to suggest to me during my interview with him on my podcast to try cryotherapy, as he swore it had dramatic effects on his post-training recovery.

I had since tried different forms of cryo chambers and had done a few cold plunges at home in the bathtub with bags of ice. This would be my first time doing it in a frozen lake.

Luckily, there were a few friendly locals there who apparently did this on a weekly basis, so we at least had people who knew what they were doing and were ready to give a few pointers. Anita decided she would take the plunge with me, and we gamely joined the group.

For some reason, all of us getting undressed to our swimwear in freezing temperatures did not seem so strange. 'Rub your skin all over to generate heat before you lower yourself in,' one of the locals suggested as she saw how pale and tentative I looked. Death from cardiac arrest or hypothermia were just some of the thoughts that were running in my head.

I slowly lowered my toes, ankles, all the way to my knees, and decided to just go for it and push off my entire body into the freezing waters. The shock from the freezing cold water put my body into sensory overload. I started to take big gasps of air as my sympathetic nervous system increased my heart rate. This was the cold shock response, and I was in full fight or flight mode.

The next thirty seconds or so seemed like an eternity. There was definitely a numbing pain I was not prepared to cope with, and I decided I'd had enough and swam back to the dock. The water, at around four degrees Celsius, was actually warmer than the air, so getting back up didn't bring any more relief from the cold. Then all of a sudden, as I was towelling off, I could feel a surge of warmth and euphoria envelop my entire being. The dopamine and endorphins were starting to kick in at full force. I, in that moment, felt like Superman.

The jetlag was gone, and I functioned for the rest of the day as if I had not even been travelling from halfway across the world for the last twenty-four hours. Why had I only discovered this crazy, superhuman ritual just now?

I would eventually take the plunge again filming in Finland a month from then, but I would do it with an expert and last in colder temperatures and stay in the water seven times longer.

When Roger Bannister broke the four-minute mile barrier in 1954, he was successful in not so much finding a new way to train but in opening the gates for a tidal wave of people who broke their own mental barrier of what was once the Holy Grail of athletic achievement. In Finland one month later, I would break my mental barrier and come out of the experience somewhat of an expert—at least, in how I am able to control my mind and body in freezing cold waters.

But a cold plunge is just the tip of the iceberg—pardon the pun—as it is just one of the many forms of biohacking that people have discovered through the years. Biohacking sounds a little dystopian—but contrary to the images of dark labs with machinery and thunder a la Victor Frankenstein, biohacking seeks to make changes to one's lifestyle, diet, or environment in order to optimize and enhance physical and mental performance. Using science, technology, and various self-experimentation methods, one can improve a myriad of aspects of human performance, health, and longevity.

Silicon Valley entrepreneur and author Dave Asprey coined the term 'biohacking' in 2012, inspiring a movement of self-experimentation and wellness practices. He defines it as:

(v): To change the environment outside of you and inside of you so you have full control of your biology, to allow you to upgrade your body, mind, and your life.

(n) The art and science of becoming superhuman.[137]

And in a way, humans have been biohacking ever since we started developing medicines and cures. From using leeches to treat skin diseases in ancient Egypt,[138] to the development of acupuncture in ancient China,[139] various medical practices and innovations were being discovered in search for cures for varying ailments of the mind and body. Almost seventy-five years ago, life expectancy was only up to 46.5 years old. By 2022, this has increased to 71.7 years. We have discovered and created some of the best nutrition humans need, the medicine to cure or at least manage most illnesses, and used technology to our advantage when it comes to developing things such as artificial organs and in general improving quality of life.

If you take a look at the aspirations of some of the billionaires, aside from space travel and setting up colonies on Mars, more and more of them seem to think that their final frontier is immortality, or at least as close to it as they can get. The XPRIZE Healthspan Competition, with an allocation of $101M, seeks to incentivize teams to develop innovative solutions that can measurably improve health and extend the functional, disease-free period of human life. This includes interventions that address age-related diseases, optimize wellness and vitality, and enhance the overall quality of life as people age. A recent medical advancement also includes the TULSA-Pro, a new prostate cancer treatment for men that destroys cancerous tissue from inside the prostate gland with ultrasound heat.[140]

Longevity Escape Velocity

We are living in the most amazing time in human history. Centenarians live at present with ease and life satisfaction, but the research for healthy life extension continues: Aside from biohacking, AI Futurist Ray Kurzweil[141] talks about Longevity Escape Velocity (LEV), or the point where technology extends your life by more than one year for every year you live. Imagine riding a bike where every now and then, you can stop to fix any problems or perhaps check your tires. The idea is, as long as you keep on fixing issues or perhaps even improving your bike, you can ride that bike forever. As long as medical advances keep outpacing the ageing process, you keep getting fixes and improvements faster than you age, allowing you to continue living a healthy life much longer than currently possible.

The concept of LEV is originally attributed to Dr Aubrey de Grey, a biomedical gerontologist and co-founder of SENS Research Foundation. It suggests that once medical interventions extend human lifespan faster than time is passing, individuals could potentially 'escape' the effects of ageing and live indefinitely. This radical idea has gained attention in anti-ageing research and futurism.

I was first introduced to the term LEV by Dr Peter Diamandis when I took the executive programme at Singularity University in Silicon Valley, of which he is executive director. Dr Diamandis, founder of the XPRIZE and named by *Times* as one of the 'World's 100 Most Influential People', shared with us how he sees the future. 'Technology buys you time. We can make time abundant,' he tells us as we tried to grasp the imminent possibilities of lifespan and health span extension.

There is of course a lot of healthy discussion about this topic, and many other pioneers and recent controversial biohackers. One such controversial character is Bryan Johnson and his $2M/ year longevity project called Blueprint, where he downs around 100 supplements a day and experiments with a dizzying array of treatments and protocols.

In this chapter, I introduce the biohacks that have come to light in recent times. Some of them I have tried (but do not necessarily endorse) in my body and mind optimization journey.

But first, we discuss a definition of terms.

Life Expectancy vs Lifespan vs Health span vs Longevity

It's important to know the differences, because yes, they have different meanings. Life expectancy is the average lifespan of a specific population. For example, life expectancy in the US is

76.4 years.[142] On the other hand lifespan is the maximum time or age a species has been observed to live, such as 122 years old for humans.[143] Health span is defined as the period where a person is healthy within their individual lifespans; a person can fall ill in youth but still live for a long time.

Longevity on the other hand is the ability to live a long life beyond the average life expectancy, or the average lifespan under ideal conditions.[144] **Our goal as peak performers is to not just live long, it's to live well for as long as we are alive.**

Is Stem Cell Therapy our Future?

Advancements in heart failure management include regenerative medicine approaches, including stem cell therapy and tissue engineering, hold significant promise for repairing damaged cardiac tissue and restoring function. [145]

Precision medicine initiatives have also gained attention and traction, aiming to tailor heart failure therapies to individuals and taking into account genetics, biomarkers, and comorbidities. Integrating AI and machine learning in heart failure management has also enabled the development of predictive models for early intervention, risk reduction, and personalized treatment recommendations.

At this point in time, only a few FDA-approved stem cell-based therapies are available. The most common such treatment is the blood stem cell transplant procedure in which blood stem cells are used to treat patients with blood cancers, like leukaemia. In this procedure, harmful cancer cells are attacked with chemotherapy, then replaced with healthy stem cells that, hopefully, proliferate and grow healthy tissue.[146]

The world awaits the approval and inconclusive results of these emerging medicines.

Most Common Biohacking Techniques

Cold therapy

Cold therapy has been one of the most used and trusted recovery and biohacking protocols that have been used by everyone from fitness and biohacking aficionados to athletes of different levels. The most notable expert Wim Hof, famously known for the Wim Hof Method, describes cold therapy as one of its pillars, along with breathing and commitment.

Depending on where in the world you are, cold therapy can also be quite accessible, since getting it can be as easy as taking a cold shower. It can also get quite complicated, pricey and advanced with cryo chambers that can lower ambient air temperature to under -160 degrees Celsius.

Overall, cold therapy can provide a range of physiological and psychological benefits, including improved circulation, reduced inflammation, enhanced immune function, metabolism, mood, energy, and recovery. Cold therapy has been used by athletes for many years to promote recovery and athletic performance. However, it's essential to approach cold exposure safely and gradually, especially for individuals with underlying health conditions or who are new to cold therapy. Consulting with a healthcare professional before starting a cold exposure regimen is advisable, especially for individuals with cardiovascular or respiratory conditions.

After a number of attempts in our ice-filled bathtub, a few cryo chamber sessions as well as a brief dip in the freezing Lake Zurich in Switzerland, I was finally able to get a proper introduction on how to successfully navigate the extreme temperature changes by cold exposure and breathwork expert Leigh Ewin.

Leigh, a native Australian who has called Finland home for close to a decade, gave me a masterclass on how to properly navigate the experience of subjecting your body to extreme temperatures. I met up with Leigh at his daily watering hole, a majestic setting amidst the frozen Baltic Sea off Espoo in Finland. We stripped to our swim shorts in -5 degree Celsius weather and made the cold walk out to a deck that stretched out around thirty metres out into the frozen ocean, with all but a small patch of water amidst a sea of ice as far as my eyes could see. He gave me as much of a brief as could be given to someone who would be doing this for the first time. Prior to this, I was able to stay less than a minute in cold water. I would feel a sense of panic once my body hits the water, causing me to gasp and try to catch my breath. This time, I was able to stay beyond three minutes. Some tips from Leigh:

- **Take your time.** He instructed me to use the metal steps to slowly lower my body—first my feet, legs, all the way until my entire torso.
- **Breathing is critical.** Think of your inhale as the gas, and your exhale as the brakes. A longer exhale will allow you to also control how your body reacts to the physiological stress.
- **Take your mind away from the discomfort.** Leigh encouraged me to look out into nature and enjoy the view.
- **Feel the warmth.** Believe it or not at some point (for me it was after the first minute), your body will start to feel warm the longer you're submerged underwater, and as you emerge from the water. This is because of the scientific concept of thermodynamics—your body temperature will start to match the temperature of the water, making it feel 'warmer' than when you initially jump in. The feeling of warmth after is due to the increase in metabolic rate as the body works to generate heat to maintain core body temperature.
- **Move after.** Following the warm feeling you get after cold exposure, do gradual movements to allow blood to flow back to your extremities. As we were filming the session, I followed Leigh as he invited me to do some slow, deliberate

martial arts-type movements as well as slow push-ups. It was like a scene straight out of a movie with the guru teaching his student the ways of the martial arts. Or in this case, the cold arts. We immortalized this moment in the documentary series *Methods to Greatness* with an epic drone shot amidst the majestic nature backdrop of Finland.

DIY cold plunge

As the name suggests, this is one of the alternatives to those interested in cold exposure but do not live near frozen lakes, rivers, or oceans. As earlier mentioned, you can reap the benefits of cold exposure from a cold shower if the water is around ten to fifteen degrees Celsius. If you live in a tropical climate like me, a cold plunge is the way to go. Putting ice in a bathtub is one way to do it. You fill the bathtub to a certain level and put enough ice to get the water down to around ten degrees. Doing this takes many steps (buying or making ice, bringing it up, and unloading the ice in the bathtub), so after I tried it a few times, I was looking for the most painless, automated way so I could do this on a regular basis without any excuses.

Chest freezer cold plunge

A do-it-yourself chest freezer cold plunge involves filling up a large enough freezer with water and letting the freezer chill the water to your desired temperature. A Wi-Fi-enabled temperature controller with a sensor that you can buy on Amazon determines if the water has reached your desired temperature and will automatically turn off the freezer. There's also the matter of filtering the water so that you don't have to replace the water constantly. This chest freezer cold plunge hack reduces excuses, preparation time, and lets you control the water to your desired exact temperature.[147] There are many DIY chest freezer cold plunge videos on YouTube, and I used a few as reference for building my own, which we set up on the balcony of our bedroom. I'm lucky that my father-in-law is quite the handyman, so I had him help me out with this one.

You may come off as a little weird and scary once you go to your favourite depot measuring if the chest freezer you're considering buying can actually fit a human body (mine is 299 litres) but you just need to take your measurements well and crouch beside the freezer to double check the size. Take note of your shoulder width to see if you'll be able to even sit squarely once you're submerged.

Of course, a simpler alternative would be your ice-filled bathtub or even those portable ice plunge recovery pods if you don't have a bathtub at home. Do what works for you and good luck with the build!

Cryotherapy chamber

Whole-body cryotherapy is a medical treatment widely used in sports medicine. Cryotherapy chambers use liquid nitrogen or refrigerated cold air to create a cold environment inside the chamber. Its main purpose for athletes is to recover from injuries, but recent studies also confirmed its anti-inflammatory, anti-analgesic, and antioxidant uses. Whole-body cryotherapy as with the cold plunge has been demonstrated to be a preventive strategy against the effects of exercise-induced inflammation and soreness.[148] I've done this a few times and with different kinds of chambers, with the temperature going down to as low as -160 degrees Celsius. I stayed inside for three minutes and the feeling after is similar but also different to what you would experience in a cold plunge.

The difference in my opinion is that in the cold plunge, there is an initial cold shock that in time, you can get used to that will allow you to stay longer. For the cryotherapy chamber, the cold you feel gradually builds up as your skin temperature goes down until you can't stand it anymore. You get what you need in three minutes, and you're done. The feeling of euphoria and warmth after is the same for both.

Sauna

The multitude of benefits that can be derived from sauna has long been studied, proven, and documented. Studies have shown that heat exposure—more specifically, sauna bathing—has been proven to improve multiple markers of cardiometabolic diseases. Sauna acts as a hormetic stressor, or the right amount of stress that challenges but doesn't fatigue the body. It has been dubbed as a practical and alternative intervention for disease prevention especially for people with high-stress occupations, like firefighters, police, military personnel, and first responders.[149]

During my visit to Finland, the sauna capital of the world where there are approximately three saunas for every five people, I've had the opportunity to take things deeper and immerse myself in Finnish sauna culture. The impressive Löyly design sauna located at the tip of the Helsinki peninsula, was a perfect introduction to just how the Finns enjoy and use the sauna as a way to not just reap health benefits, but to actually integrate the activity into their social fabric. I found out that it's actually quite common to do sauna bathing as a way that families and co-workers spend time bonding. Visitors in Finland, whether for business or tourism, are usually introduced to the experience and are made to understand and appreciate that going to the sauna is a way of life for the Finns.

After the cold exposure session with Leigh Ewin, he took me to a majestic little private sauna situated just off the river within the Nuuksio National Park. We ended up doing a sauna-cold exposure protocol where we would do the sauna, lower ourselves in to cold lake water, and go back to the sauna.

Some tips from Leigh:

- In a dry sauna, make sure you put water to give off steam.
- Keep your feet up so that your legs also get the benefits since the air is colder the lower you are in the sauna. Cross your legs.

- Meditate, and give this still time for yourself.
- Breathe. In the sauna, it's ok to breathe through your mouth as the warm air can get too much for the nose to take in.
- Allow the heat to give you a warm embrace.

I've been undergoing religious sauna sessions at home for over three years now, when it just made sense for us to install one in our house so we can reap all of the health benefits. I will do an average of at least two to three sessions a week, usually after a gym workout. It's been shown that two to three sessions of sauna for no more than fifteen to twenty minutes at a time can help in post-workout relaxation and muscle recovery.[150] Personally, I feel so relaxed and calm after, and it's done wonders for my sleep. Alternating a sauna cold exposure protocol takes things to the next level, though it also consumes a lot of time. Remember to always hydrate, and you should be good.

Biohacking and Hackstacking

Much like Dave Asprey, illnesses and chronic issues that plagued Eli Abela in her youth eventually led to her becoming one of the biohacking pioneers in the Philippines as well as a human potential and vitality coach.

> If you think about it, biohacking is kind of young, but because of its explosive nature, people have really picked up the concept and started doing it on themselves. Self-experimentation is at the heart of biohacking. It's now become an explosive movement.

While it sounds intimidating, Eli shares that biohacking can involve simple practices like fasting or cold showers to advanced clinical-grade machines for addressing conditions like cancer and inflammation.

Eli eventually opened a biohacking recovery centre in
the Philippines, offering clinical-grade treatments for various
demographics, from aesthetics to mental health and wellness:

> What I wanted to do was to give people an option or an alternative
> to whatever we have out there right now, which is the medical
> paradigm conventional medicine or holistic alternative medicine,
> which can be expensive. I wanted to fill in the missing gap there
> and provide people with a different kind of treatment, different
> kind of choice.

According to Eli, biohacking can begin with something as simple as
taking in sunrise and sunset, which offers natural healing for various
ailments. Specific biohacking techniques such as oxygen training
on the other hand enhances cognitive and physical performance.
She advocates for biohacking as a tool for optimizing cellular
mechanisms and overall well-being.

For my visit with Eli, she decided that what was best for me was
called brain training, which she describes:

> With brain training with clinical grade neuroptimal neurofeedback,
> it allows you to stay flexible and resilient. So, it's training in staying
> present. So instead of mulling about, "Oh, something's going to
> happen," some sort of anticipatory anxiety, you can stay present,
> you stay in the moment, and you become your best version, no
> matter what.

This next section discusses the latest biohacking techniques and
machinery that I have personally tried out.

Biohacking Machines and Tools

These are the machines I tried out in Eli's biohacking and recovery
centre, which I used as I was recovering from my injury and

preparing for my competition. Some of them I 'hackstacked' (simply meaning practising or using multiple hacks at the same time) and did simultaneously to save on time:

Neurofeedback

Neurofeedback (the brain machine) claims to allow the brain to build flexibility and resilience with every session. 'The software feeds back information of its own dysregulated activity (called a flutter) and allows the brain to self-organize,' shares Eli. The feedback is auditory—usually they are differently timed clicks or gaps that occur during a movie that you watch or audio that you listen to. Over time, the brain knows itself so much so that it organizes itself even before the flutter happens. Each brain will have its own unique flutter, and the important thing is that it's your own brain that does the balancing, and not the machine. What that means: people can find sleep again after the brain balances and quiets down, people are less reactive and more proactive, they have greater patience and tolerance, they give in less to addictive behaviour, they are more energized, bad habits or nervous ticks diminish, anxiety lessens.

PEMF Mat with NanoVi®

A PEMF Mat provides low frequency pulsed magnetic fields to stimulate energy production within cells or injured areas.[151] Users lay down or sit on the mat, which is also combined with NanoVi® technology, developed to supplement the body with the same signal that it makes naturally to signal cells to repair themselves. The mat is recommended for injured athletes or those who seek to reduce inflammation in their bodies.[152]

RedBed

The RedBed uses red light therapy (RLT) for treating wrinkles, redness, acne, scars and other signs of ageing.[153] It is said to help in sleep, where most cellular repair and detox happens.

CAROL Bike

With the claim of being 'The bike that gets you fittest, fastest,' the CAROL Bike is a commercial-grade exercise bike optimized for Reduced Exertion HIIT (REHIT). The machine features twenty AI-guided, workouts and fitness tests.[154] It aims to deliver superior health and fitness benefits in 90 per cent less time compared to regular cardio.

Exercise with oxygen therapy (EWOT)

Using an oxygen system concentrator, EWOT involves breathing higher levels of oxygen during exercise. It is said that this can increase strength, endurance, and stamina, and an overall more effective workout in the same time frame. This oxygen therapy also improves blood flow and circulation.[155]

Compression therapy

Compression therapy for lymphatic drainage involves using specialized compression garments. These garments apply controlled pressure to the affected area, promoting the movement of lymphatic fluid, reducing swelling, and supporting lymphatic function. It promotes circulation and decreases pain and soreness brought about by delayed onset muscle soreness or DOMS. It's also a good way to warm up before training as well as a post-workout protocol.

The times I used this felt really good, and was akin to getting a massage as the pressure helped alleviate the lactic acid buildup in my legs.

Hyperbaric oxygen therapy

Hyperbaric Oxygen Therapy or HBOT is a medical treatment that involves breathing pure oxygen in a pressurized chamber or room. During HBOT sessions, the atmospheric pressure is increased to levels higher than normal, allowing the lungs to absorb more oxygen than would be possible at standard atmospheric pressure.

Originally used in the treatment of decompression sickness or 'the bends' experienced by scuba divers, HBOT's additional therapeutic benefits of increased oxygen concentration in the bloodstream led to usage for other treatments such as support for healing and recovery processes, reduction of inflammation in injured or damaged tissues, and the management of other medical conditions.

I've tried HBOT a few times, from the small soft-sided portable capsule chambers to the big chamber versions that can accommodate a dozen patients and where you breathe 100 per cent pure oxygen. There is definitely a big difference in pressure capacity between the two. The science makes sense, but I suggest you do further research before trying HBOT as cost and time considerations are substantial and it is a big commitment if you really aim to achieve long-term results.

Sensory deprivation tank

A sensory deprivation tank, also known as a flotation tank or isolation tank, is a soundproof and lightproof chamber filled with a solution of water and Epsom salts, creating a buoyant environment in which individuals can float effortlessly.

The purpose of a deprivation tank is to provide an environment of sensory isolation, minimizing external stimuli such as light, sound, and gravity. This sensory deprivation is thought to induce a state of deep relaxation and promote mental and physical well-being.

People typically lie down in the tank, floating effortlessly on the surface of the water, which is heated to skin temperature to minimize sensory input. The tank is enclosed to block out external noise and light, creating a serene and tranquil environment.

Floating in the tank reminded me of the time when I took a dip in the Dead Sea as the Epsom salts make you buoyant so you can float effortlessly. It's a cool, trippy experience, though not really a biohacking protocol I would do on a regular basis.

Everyday Biohacking

Biohacking doesn't have to be complicated (or expensive) when incorporating them into your everyday life. Try out the following techniques and see the benefits yourself:

Table 7.1: Biohacking techniques

Technique	How-To	Benefits
Sunlight exposure	The best time to get sun exposure is early in the morning which also helps set an internal timer for the body.	For Caucasians, a half-hour in the summer sun in a bathing suit can initiate the release of 50,000 IU (1.25 mg) vitamin D into the circulation within twenty-four hours of exposure; this same amount of exposure yields 20,000–30,000 IU in tanned individuals and 8,000–10,000 IU in dark-skinned people.[156]
Time in nature	Two hours a week in nature is ideal to report good health and psychological well-being.[157]	Nature has been found to have robust effects on people's health—physically, mentally, and emotionally. It can lower blood pressure and stress hormone levels, reduce nervous system arousal, enhance immune system function, increase self-esteem, reduce anxiety, and improve mood.
Sleep	From power naps to a consistent sleep cycle, tracking and getting a good amount of sleep every night is ideal	Find out more about the full benefits of sleep in Chapter 1.
Movement	Make time to move at least thirty minutes a day or 180 minutes a week	Find out more about the full benefits of movement in Chapter 3.

Your to-do list to incorporate biohacks for peak performance:

- Which of these biohacks interested you the most? **List down your top three**—and commit to trying out at least one of them and see where it gets you and if you can commit to doing this long-term.
- Overwhelmed? **Try narrowing down your improvement priorities**: e.g. you may want to improve your sleep. From this, choose the biohack that fits your goal the best and monitor/measure how that biohack helps you.
- Don't have the time? That's always the most convenient excuse. **Get a partner to join you in trying something out.** Look for the easiest biohack that you can incorporate within your day and try them out with a partner who will commit with you, and you can be accountable to.

Epilogue

'You're not going to push ahead when it's someone else's mission.
It needs to be yours.'

—*Peter H. Diamandis*, Bold: How to Go Big,
Create Wealth and Impact the World

If you had an opportunity to become the best version of yourself, would you do whatever it takes to become it?

Sleep, nutrition, movement: it's really quite funny how our perceived childhood punishments have become our adult goals. 'Go to bed early! Eat your vegetables! Squat in the corner for five minutes!' And yet forming these habits and making them a consistent part of our lives takes a lot of work and unwavering commitment. When life gets in the way, how do we get ourselves back on track? Picking up a new habit is easy. Maintaining it for life is the million-dollar question.

When I first set out to write this book, the intention was clear: to distill the performance protocols and mindset of the very best peak performers, experts, and coaches from across the globe.

The book would also be one big experiment. One that I had given myself both an excuse and permission to subject my mind and body to at this age and stage of my life.

I've also realized through the course of writing this book that this along with other things I've done the past few years are a direct manifestation of a midlife crisis. Writing a new bucket list, wanting to compete again and become part of my country's national team, biohacking to try to delay the inevitable sarcopenia and mental decline that follows with ageing.

That's why the concept of LEV or longevity escape velocity appeals so much to me. The potential of lifestyle choices, technology, and medical interventions playing a role in extending health span and not just lifespan is now a primordial concern. Have I really lived more than half my life already? What lies in store for me for the next half and how can I maintain my physical and mental faculties?

It's not the getting older part I'm worried about. It's getting older and not being able to do the things I want to do and having a quality of life free from pain and disease. I want a long life, not just for myself but for my wife and family. I want to be there for our future grandchildren and be able to play with them and travel and stick around for a long time. Just like the Professor of Happiness, Markku Ojanen. I strongly suspect I'm not the only one who aspires for this and wants to do something about it.

All around us, there are people who are severely unprepared for old age. The concerns and pursuits of career, family, and other priorities have relegated our mental and physical health to the back seat. The journey to our best life and a healthy life at old age ideally begins as early as childhood and is a lifelong commitment.

Dr Peter Diamandis posed a question to me five years ago: 'What is your massively transformative purpose?' It was a life-changing question that made me want to find my true purpose in this world.

He posited, 'The world's biggest problems are the world's biggest opportunities. You are massively empowered. What are you going to do with it?'

What if . . .

I could channel all this knowledge, passion and purpose into something that allows people to live their best lives? If we begin the right habits early, we set ourselves up for life. But we can't do this alone. We need a community, a tribe that will support us on this journey.

What was unclear when I first started writing this book were the deeper reasons for putting this out into the world. What did I want to achieve? What was the message that I wanted to convey? What result was I going for? It's now become clear that this journey that I started should be a journey that others can eventually take themselves.

The Science

We'll begin with science, and technology. We will in the near future develop a platform that allows us to break through the noise and clutter and aggregate the essential information and resources to live our best lives. Sleep. Nutrition and supplementation. Movement and exercise. Mental health and brain optimization. Injury and disease prevention and intervention. Biohacking and Longevity. We will create programmes that allow people to gain access to the things they need for their health and wellness journey.

Every person is different. We have different needs, predispositions, and goals. We must leverage technology to find the most suitable solution for each person based on their unique circumstances and objectives. We can only inspire them to a point. At the end of the day, they're not going to push ahead when it's someone else's mission. It needs to be theirs.

The Art

The Art is the challenging part. How do we get the best experts, companies and communities to be part of the platform? Remember the *Methods to Greatness* documentary series that I was talking about? The first season of that had me travelling the world and collaborating with experts and companies and testing out the methods, protocols, products and services that allow one to achieve peak performance and live their best lives. For the subsequent seasons, I bring in others who will take their own health and optimization journey as well. If they stick to the programme where we create specific, measurable, achievable, relevant, and time-bound goals that they actually achieve, others will want to follow suit.

We'll film everything in the documentary of how to get people to take a life transformative health and wellness journey using our platform and community. As we do this, we also document and show how we build a health tech startup from the ground up. This would be the platform's secret sauce and unfair advantage. The documentary series feeds into the startup and vice versa.

We need to be having conversations with companies and partnering with them to improve the lives of their employees and teams. We also need to involve the different tribes and communities that will be the platform's support system. If we're able to start strong with a clear focus and deliver quantifiable results, the rest of the business in time will grow so that we can eventually democratize access not just for companies but to as many people as possible.

Peter Diamandis says that 'Right now, and for the first time ever, a passionate and committed individual has access to the technology, minds, and capital required to take on any challenge.' I believe the time is now to do something that's never been done before in the health and wellness space.

I invite you to be part of our community by visiting MethodstoGreatness.com

Acknowledgements

To my father Dave, thank you for all the times you took me to those tennis clinics when I was eleven years old that started me on my fitness journey. To my wife Monica, thank you for being my lifelong partner and co-conspirator both mentally and physically. Danielle, Luis and David. Your mom and I look forward to sticking around long enough so we can make many more memories together.

Thank you to our team at Streetpark Productions Inc. and Dragon's Nest. Leng, as always for your support for what is now our fourth book. Don, Eugene, Jun, LJ for journeying with me on *Methods to Greatness* and for supporting this book project as well. To my writing and research team Annelle and Vanessa, this was a herculean effort, but we pulled it off.

To all my interviewees and collaborators from around the world, thank you for sharing your knowledge, experience and expertise.

Bobby Macasaet, Sean Argos and Archie Rillo, Ed Sediego, Carlo Buzzichelli, Gary Cablayan, Dr. Gar Eufemio, Celine Fürst, Sofia Santelices, Kent Primor, Christine Fajardo, Anita Berardi, Ambassador Pyykkö Juha, Veera Kaarela, Mikael Malmivaara, Sara Jäntti, Prof. Helene Patounas, Eli Abela, Janne Kallio,Pekka Pohjakallio, Dr Xiaoran Liu, Mitch Genato, Linus Reyes, Kristine Santos, Patrizia Usala, Kevin Donogue, Dr Luis Reyes, Jyrki Lee-Korhonen, Dr Fabio Valoppi, Cathy Turvill, Jasmine Goh, Matti Kontsas, Scott Larsen, JayR Felix, Toby Claudio, Luis Gatmaitan, Mark Cristi, Abbie Pua, Alexandre Vessella, Marvin Navarro, Nameeta Dargani, Gurudev Sri Sri Ravishankar, Victor Antonio,

Leigh Ewin, Miki Vuorisalmi, Erwin Valencia, Dr Burcu Demiray, Andrew De Castro, Sayaka De Castro, Azuma, Pia Wurtzbach, Jose 'Jomag' Magsaysay, Markku Ojanen, Dr Jun Rafanan, Maris Torres-Sunang, Dado Hipolito, Jörg-Michael Rupp, Dr Tewis Bouwmeester, Dr Ann Earts, Janne Pylväs.

References

1   Eric Suni and Kimberley Truong, '100+ Sleep Statistics', *Sleep Foundation*, September 26, 2023. https://www.sleepfoundation.org/how-sleep-works/sleep-facts-statistics

2   'Sleep Statistics and Facts', *NCOA Adviser*, March 11, 2024, https://www.ncoa.org/adviser/sleep/sleep-statistics/.

3   National Institute of General Medical Sciences (NIGMS), 'National Institute of General Medical Sciences', n.d. https://www.nigms.nih.gov/education/fact-sheets/Pages/circadian-rhythms.aspx

4   Matt Walker, 'A Walk Through the Stages of Sleep', n.d. https://www.ted.com/talks/matt_walker_a_walk_through_the_stages_of_sleep?subtitle=en

5   Andrew Huberman, 'Dr. Matt Walker: The Science & Practice of Perfecting Your Sleep', April 16, 2024, https://www.hubermanlab.com/episode/dr-matthew-walker-the-science-and-practice-of-perfecting-your-sleep.

6   Jay Summer and Abhinav Singh, 'Can You Die from Not Sleeping?', *Sleep Foundation*, May 11, 2023, https://www.sleepfoundation.org/sleep-faqs/can-you-die-from-not-sleeping#references-207800.

7   Huberman Lab, 'About Dr. Andrew Huberman', n.d. https://www.hubermanlab.com/about.

8   Andrew Huberman, 'Sleep Toolkit: Tools for Optimizing Sleep & Sleep-Wake Timing', August 7, 2022. https://www.hubermanlab.com/episode/sleep-toolkit-tools-for-optimizing-sleep-and-sleep-wake-timing

9   Andrew Huberman, 'Maximizing Productivity, Physical & Mental Health with Daily Tools', July 11, 2021, https://www.hubermanlab.com/episode/maximizing-productivity-physical-and-mental-health-with-daily-tools.

10 Andrew Huberman, 'Optimize Your Learning & Creativity with Science-based Tools', February 21, 2021, https://www.hubermanlab.com/episode/optimize-your-learning-and-creativity-with-science-based-tools.

11 Brendon Burchard, 'Sleep Better: My Evening Routine - Brendon Burchard', *Brendon Burchard*, May 19, 2020, https://brendon.com/blog/my-evening-routine/.

12 Sleep Foundation, 'Blue Light: What It Is and How It Affects Sleep', January 12, 2024, https://www.sleepfoundation.org/bedroom-environment/blue-light#:~:text=Being%20exposed%20to%20blue%20light,to%20many%20negative%20health%20impacts.

13 Lucy Bryan, 'Alcohol and Sleep', *Sleep Foundation*, May 7, 2024, https://www.sleepfoundation.org/nutrition/alcohol-and-sleep.

14 Jay Summer and Dr Abhinav Singh. 'Napping: Benefits and Tips', *Sleep Foundation*, March 11, 2024, https://www.sleepfoundation.org/napping.

15 CredibleMind. 'CredibleMind', n.d. https://ihscm.crediblemind.com/podcasts/naps-with-matthew-walker?utm_source=email&utm_campaign=CM_resourceroundup.

16 'The Benefits of Napping', *National Sleep Foundation*, December 22, 2022, https://www.thensf.org/the-benefits-of-napping/.

17 Lomas, Emilina. 'How Long Is a Nap Ideally?', *The Pulse Blog*, July 9, 2024, https://ouraring.com/blog/how-long-should-you-nap/.

18 Ryan, Tom, PhD. 'Sleep in the Military', *Sleep Foundation*, July 11, 2023, https://www.sleepfoundation.org/sleep-in-the-military.

19 Arnal, Pierrick J., et al., 'Benefits of Sleep Extension on Sustained Attention and Sleep Pressure Before and During Total Sleep Deprivation and Recovery', *SLEEP* 38, no. 12: 1935–43 (2015), https://doi.org/10.5665/sleep.5244.

20 Tim Ferriss, 'Performance Coach Andy Galpin — Rebooting Tim's Sleep, Nutrition, Supplements, and Training for 2024', January 18, 2024, https://www.youtube.com/watch?v=gS4eU1LJeUU.

21 Cheri D. Mah et al., 'The Effects of Sleep Extension on the Athletic Performance of Collegiate Basketball Players', *Sleep*, 34. 943-50 (2011), 10.5665/SLEEP.1132.

22 Oura Team. 'Your Oura Readiness Score', February 7, 2024, https://ouraring.com/blog/readiness-score/.

23 Shalini Paruthi, et al., 'Recommended Amount of Sleep for Pediatric Populations: A Consensus Statement of the American Academy of Sleep Medicine', *Journal of Clinical Sleep Medicine*, 12(6):785–786 (2016), https://doi.org/10.5664/jcsm.5866.

24 Consensus Conference Panel, Nathaniel F. Watson, M. Safwan Badr, et al., 'Recommended Amount of Sleep for A Healthy Adult: A Joint Consensus Statement of the American Academy of Sleep Medicine and Sleep Research Society', *Journal of Clinical Sleep Medicine*,11(6):591–592 (2015), https://doi.org/10.5664/jcsm.4758.

25 Yuval Noah Harari. *Sapiens: A Brief History of Humankind.* New York: Harper Perennial, 2015.

26 Lauri Reuter, 'The Future of Food | SingularityU Nordic Summit', January 9, 2019. https://www.youtube.com/watch?v=KT0iKdBXmwg

27 Kearney J. 'Food consumption trends and drivers', *Philosophical transactions of the Royal Society of London. Series B, Biological sciences*, 365(1554): 2793–807 (2010). doi:10.1098/rstb.2010.0149.

28 John Hopkins Medicine, 'Grapefruit Benefits', https://www.hopkinsmedicine.org/health/wellness-and-prevention/grapefruit-benefits.

29 Esther Ellis, 'Staying Away from Fad Diets', March 18, 2019, https://www.eatright.org/health/wellness/diet-trends/staying-away-from-fad-diets.

30 AiazaTahreem, et al., 'Fad Diets: Facts and Fiction', *Frontiers in Nutrition*, 9:960922 (2022), doi:10.3389/fnut.2022.960922.

31 Harvard T.H. Chan School of Public Health, The Nutrition Source. 'Diet Review: Paleo Diet for Weight Loss', last reviewed 2022. https://nutritionsource.hsph.harvard.edu/healthy-weight/diet-reviews/paleo-diet/.

32 Harvard T.H. Chan School of Public Health, The Nutrition Source, 'Diet Review: The Ketogenic Diet for Weight Loss', last reviewed 2022. https://nutritionsource.hsph.harvard.edu/healthy-weight/diet-reviews/ketogenic-diet/.

33 Robby Berman, 'Vegan vs omnivorous diet: Which is more effective for weight loss?', December 11, 2023. https://www.medicalnewstoday.com/articles/vegan-vs-omnivorous-diet-which-is-more-effective-weight-loss#What-makes-a-healthy-plant-based-diet.

34 World Health Organisation (WHO), 'Intervention: Increasing fruit and vegetable consumption to reduce the risk of noncommunicable diseases', August 9, 2023, https://www.who.int/tools/elena/interventions/fruit-vegetables-ncds.

35 Daljeet Singh Dhanjal et al., 'Plant Fortification of the Diet for Anti-Ageing Effects: A Review', *Nutrients*, 12(10): 3008, (2020), https://doi.org/10.3390/nu12103008.

36 Milly Ryan-Harshman, and Walid Aldoori, 'New dietary reference intakes for macronutrients and fibre', *Canadian family physician Medecin de famille canadien*, 52(2):177–9 (2006), https://www.ncbi.nlm.nih.gov/pmc/articles/PMC1479724/#:~:text=Dietary%20reference%20intakes%20suggest%20that,%25%20to%2035%25%20from%20protein.

37 National Institute of Health, 'Dietary Supplement Fact Sheets', https://ods.od.nih.gov/factsheets/list-all/.

38 Giovanni Savarino et al., 'Macronutrient balance and micronutrient amounts through growth and development.' *Italian Journal of Pediatrics*, 47(1):109 (2021), doi:10.1186/s13052-021-01061-0.

39 The Institute For Functional Medicine, 'Eating for Your Microbiome', The Institute For Functional Medicine, https://drrobart.com/wp-content/uploads/Eating-For-Your-Microbiome.pdf.

40 Cleveland Clinic, 'Gut Microbiome', last reviewed on August 18, 2023, https://my.clevelandclinic.org/health/body/25201-gut-microbiome.

41 Birgitte Svennevig, 'Intermittent fasting itself will not make your extra kilos disappear', *University of Southern Denmark*, January 2, 2024, https://www.sdu.dk/en/om-sdu/fakulteterne/naturvidenskab/nyheder-2024/ketosis.

42 Philip M.M. Ruppert et al, 'Mechanisms of hepatic fatty acid oxidation and ketogenesis during fasting', *Trends in Endocrinology & Metabolism TEM*, 35(2):107–124 (2024), doi:10.1016/j.tem.2023.10.002.

43 Thomas DeLauer, 'Why Dr. Peter Attia Changed his Mind on Fasting (and 4 other Longevity Topics)', May13, 2023, https://www.youtube.com/watch?v=Tb6gMegtLcg.

44 Kenneth Vitale and Andrew Getzin, 'Nutrition and Supplement Update for the Endurance Athlete: Review and Recommendations', *Nutrients*,11(6):1289 (2019). doi: 10.3390/nu11061289.

45 Yijia Zhang et al., 'Can Magnesium Enhance Exercise Performance?', *Nutrients*, 9(9):946 (2017). doi: 10.3390/nu9090946.

46 Louisa Richards, '30 muscle-building foods to fuel your goals', March 31, 2021, https://www.medicalnewstoday.com/articles/muscle-building-foods#importance-of-nutrition.

47 Diego A Bonilla et al., 'The 4R's Framework of Nutritional Strategies for Post-Exercise Recovery: A Review with Emphasis on New Generation of Carbohydrates.' *International Journal of Environmental Research and Public Health*, 18(1) (2020), doi:10.3390/ijerph18010103.

48 Kamil Rodak et al., 'Caffeine as a Factor Influencing the Functioning of the Human Body-Friend or Foe?', *Nutrients*, 13(9):3088 (2021), doi: 10.3390/nu13093088.

49 Danielle Pacheco and Dr Dustin Cotliar, 'Caffeine and Sleep.' *Sleep Foundation*, April 17, 2024, https://www.sleepfoundation.org/nutrition/caffeine-and-sleep.

50 Salehi B, Mishra AP, Nigam M, Sener B, Kilic M, Sharifi-Rad M, Fokou PVT, Martins N, Sharifi-Rad J. "Resveratrol: A Double-Edged Sword in Health Benefits." Biomedicines. 2018 Sep 9;6(3):91. doi: 10.3390/biomedicines6030091.

51 World Health Organisation, 'No level of alcohol consumption is safe for our health', January 4, 2023, https://www.who.int/europe/news/item/04-01-2023-no-level-of-alcohol-consumption-is-safe-for-our-health.

52 Harvard Medical School, 'Diet rich in resveratrol offers no health boost', *Harvard Health Publishing*, May 15, 2014, https://www.health.harvard.edu/blog/diet-rich-resveratrol-offers-health-boost-201405157153.

53 Oura Team, 'What is Heart Rate Variability (HRV)?', September 20, 2023, https://ouraring.com/blog/what-is-heart-rate-variability/.

54 World Health Organisation, 'Health Diet', April 29, 2020, https://www.who.int/news-room/fact-sheets/detail/healthy-diet.

55 Department of Science and Technology, 'Pinggang Pinoy: Healthy food plate for Filipinos', *Food and Nutrition Research institute*, https://fnri.dost.gov.ph/index.php/116-pinggang-pinoy.

56 Harvard T.H. Chan School of Public Health, 'Diet Review: MIND Diet', *The Nutrition Source*, last reviewed August 2023, https://nutritionsource.hsph.harvard.edu/healthy-weight/diet-reviews/mind-diet/.

57 Jennifer Falbe, et al., 'Potentially addictive properties of sugar-sweetened beverages among adolescents', *Appetite*, 133:130–137 (2019), doi: 10.1016/j.appet.2018.10.032.

58 Catherine Brillantes-Turvill, *Turn Back Time: Natural Anti-Aging Choices* (Sorrell Publishing Company, 2012).

59 Office of Dietary Supplements, 'Omega-3 Fatty Acids', *National Institutes of Health*, updated July 18, 2022, https://ods.od.nih.gov/factsheets/Omega3FattyAcids-Consumer/.

60 Jacob Dunn and Michael H. Grider, 'Physiology, Adenosine Triphosphate', *National Library of Medicine*, updated February 13, 2023, https://www.ncbi.nlm.nih.gov/books/NBK553175/.

61 Darren G. Candow et al., '"Heads Up" for Creatine Supplementation and its Potential Applications for Brain Health and Function', *Sports Med* 53 (Suppl 1):49–65 (2023), https://doi.org/10.1007/s40279-023-01870-9.

62 Melvin Williams, 'Dietary supplements and sports performance: herbals', *Journal of the International Society of Sports Nutrition*, 3:1, 1–6 (2006), doi:10.1186/1550-2783-3-1-1.

63 Dirk W. Luchtman and Cai Song, 'Cognitive enhancement by omega-3 fatty acids from child-hood to old age: Findings from animal and clinical studies', *Neuropharmacology*, 64:550–565 (2013), https://doi.org/10.1016/j.neuropharm.2012.07.019.

64 Matěj Malík and Pavel Tlustoš, 'Nootropics as Cognitive Enhancers: Types, Dosage and Side Effects of Smart Drugs', *Nutrients*, 14(16):3367 (2022), doi: 10.3390/nu14163367.

65 Cleveland Clinic, 'Adaptogens', last reviewed in 2022, https://my.clevelandclinic.org/health/drugs/22361-adaptogens.

66 Jennifer Berry, 'What are nootropics (smart drugs)?', *Medical News Today*, September 19, 2019, https://www.medicalnewstoday.com/articles/326379.

67 Huberman Lab, 'Sleep Toolkit: Tools for Optimizing Sleep & Sleep-Wake Timing', August 7, 2022, https://www.hubermanlab.com/episode/sleep-toolkit-tools-for-optimizing-sleep-and-sleep-wake-timing.

68 Kaori Yokoi-Shimizu et al., 'Effect of Docosahexaenoic Acid and Eicosapentaenoic Acid Supplementation on Sleep Quality in Healthy Subjects: A Randomized, Double-Blinded, Placebo-Controlled Trial', *Nutrients*, 14 (19): 4136 (2022), doi:10.3390/nu14194136.

69 Dr Elisabeth Roider et al., *The Maximon Longevity Compendium: A Practical Guide to Extending Your Healthy Lifespan* (Maximon—The Longevity Company Builder, 2023).

70 OECD, 'Dispelling "Neuromyths"', *Understanding the Brain: The Birth of a Learning Science*, 107-126, June 12, 2007. https://doi.org/10.1787/9789264029132-9-en

71 Ashley Beckwith and Emma Parkhurst, 'The Mental Benefits of Decluttering', *Utah State University, Mental Health Education Extension*, July 1, 2022, https://extension.usu.edu/mentalhealth/articles/the-mental-benefits-of-decluttering.

72 NHS UK, 'Bouncing back from life's challenges', *Better Health: Every Mind Matters*, https://www.nhs.uk/every-mind-matters/mental-wellbeing-tips/self-help-cbt-techniques/bouncing-back-from-lifes-challenges/.

73 Nansook Park et al, 'Positive Psychology and Physical Health: Research and Applications', *American journal of lifestyle medicine*, 10(3) 200–206 (2014), doi:10.1177/1559827614550277.

74 AQAI, 'The AQ Model', https://www.aqai.io/resources/the-aq-model.

75 Nancy Giordano, 'Leadering: Why Visionary Leaders Are Investing In Adaptability Quotient', *Medium*, June 7, 2022, https://nancygiordano.medium.com/leadering-why-visionary-leaders-are-investing-in-adaptability-quotient-fe838ee2c1d3.

76 SBS-ED, 'How to improve your AQ and become more adaptable', *Stellenbosch Business School, Executive Development*, November 26, 2019, https://sbs-ed.com/how-to-improve-your-aq-and-become-more-adaptable/.

77 American Psychological Association, 'Stress effects on the body', March 8, 2023, https://www.apa.org/topics/stress/body.

78 Michael Fredric Roizen, *The RealAge® Makeover* (HarperCollins Publishers Inc, 1999, 2004).

79 'Coping With Stress', Centre for Disease and Control Prevention, October 2, 2015, http://medbox.iiab.me/modules/en-cdc/www.cdc.gov/violenceprevention/pub/coping_with_stress_tips.html.

80 Bronwyn Fryer, 'Storytelling That Moves People', *Harvard Business Review*, 2003, https://hbr.org/2003/06/storytelling-that-moves-people.

81 Victor Antonio, 16:07 of meeting notes, January 17, 2024. https://otter.ai/u/7ultQkQ-niOWTFoRFXgR7Bf0T9s?t=967s&tab=summary.

82 American Psychological Association, 'Mindfulness', *APA Dictionary of Psychology*, https://www.apa.org/topics/mindfulness.

83   National Center for Complementary and Integrative Health, 'Yoga: Effectiveness and Safety', last updated August 2023, https://www. nccih.nih.gov/health/yoga-effectiveness-and-safety.

84   Dr Ishwar V. Basavaraddi, 'Yoga History', *Ministry of Ayush, Government of India*, https://yoga.ayush.gov.in/Yoga-History/.

85   Denise Everheart, 'Guided Meditation: Help for Anxiety, Stress, Sleep, and More', *The Art of Living*.

86   American Psychological Association, 'Mindfulness', *APA Dictionary of Psychology*, https://www.apa.org/topics/mindfulness.

87   Chris Williams, 'Mindfulness vs Grounding—What's The Difference?', *Heartland Therapy Connection*, December 20, 2022, https:// heartlandtherapyconnection.com/mindfulness-vs-grounding/.

88   Tchiki Davis, 'Manifestation: Definition, Meaning, and How to Do It', *The Berkeley Well-Being Institute*, https://www.berkeleywellbeing. com/manifestation.html.

89   Student Voices, 'Erwin Bendedict Valencia', *Penn LPS Online*, https:// lpsonline.sas.upenn.edu/about-penn-lps-online/student-voices/ erwin-benedict-valencia.

90   Positive Psychology Center, 'PERMA™ Theory of Well-Being and PERMA™ Workshops', *Penn Arts & Sciences*, https://ppc.sas.upenn. edu/learn-more/perma-theory-well-being-and-perma-workshops.

91   Martin Seligman, 'PERMA and the building blocks of well being', *The Journal of Positive Psychology*, 13 (4):1–3. February, 2018.

92   Felix Richter, 'Charted: How life expectancy is changing around the world', *World Economic Forum*, February 23, 2023, https://www. weforum.org/agenda/2023/02/charted-how-life-expectancy-is-changing-around-the-world/.

93   Kokoro Shirai, 'Social Determinants of Health on the Island of Okinawa', in *Health in Japan: Social Epidemiology of Japan since the 1964 Tokyo Olympics* edited by Eric Brunner, Noriko Cable, and Hiroyasu Iso (Oxford, 2020; online edn, Oxford Academic, 22 Oct. 2020), https://doi.org/10.1093/oso/9780198848134.003.0019.

94   World Health Organization, 'Mental Disorders', June 8, 2022.

95   Press Centre, 'Pia Alonzo Wurtzbach, UNAIDS Goodwill Ambassador for Asia and the Pacific', *UNAIDS*, May 3, 2017, https://www.unaids.org/en/aboutunaids/unaidsambassadors/pia-alonzo-wurtzbach.

96   John F. Helliwell et al., 'World Happiness, Trust and Social Connections in Times of Crisis', in *World Happiness Report 2023*, 11th ed., Chapter 2.

97   Guendalina Bastioli and Margaret E. Rice, 'Exercise Boosts Dopamine Release and this Requires Brain-Derived Neurotrophic Factor', *Journal Club 2022 Articles, NYU Grossman School of Medicine*, https://med.nyu.edu/departments-institutes/neuroscience/research/journal-club/journal-club-2022-articles/exercise-boosts-dopamine-release-this-requires-bdnf.

98   Joseph J. Knapik, 'The importance of physical fitness for injury prevention: part 1', *Journal of special operations medicine: a peer reviewed journal for SOF medical professionals*,15(1):123–7 (2015), https://pubmed.ncbi.nlm.nih.gov/25770810/.

99   Health Topics, 'Sports Injuries', *National Institute of Arthritis and Musculoskeletal and Skin Diseases*, last reviewed September 2024, https://www.niams.nih.gov/health-topics/sports-injuries.

100   Shona L. Halsen, 'Recovery Techniques for Athletes', *Sports Science Exchange, Gatorade Sports Science Institute*, January 2014, https://www.gssiweb.org/sports-science-exchange/article/sse-120-recovery-techniques-for-athletes.

101   Emily Abbate, 'How Making Time for Active Recovery Will Boost Your Workouts', *Men's Health*, March 15, 2019, https://www.menshealth.com/fitness/a26827583/active-recovery/.

102   Ortiz, Robert O Jr et al., 'A Systematic Review on the Effectiveness of Active Recovery Interventions on Athletic Performance of Professional-, Collegiate-, and Competitive-Level Adult Athletes', *Journal of strength and conditioning research*, 33(8):2275–2287 (2019), doi:10.1519/JSC.0000000000002589.

103   Cord Life: Umbilical Cord Blood and Cord Lining Banking, https://www.cordlife.ph/en/discover-cord-banking?gad_source=1&gclid=EAIaIQobChMIq7ujkouwhQMVZKVmAh3xag7aEAAYASAAEgI5SfD_BwE.

104   Kathryn Whitbourne, 'Should You Bank Your Baby's Cord Blood?', *Grow by WebMD*, March 17, 2023, https://www.webmd.com/baby/should-you-bank-your-babys-cord-blood.

105   Word Health Organization, 'The Top 10 Causes of Death', August 7, 2023, https://www.who.int/news-room/fact-sheets/detail/the-top-10-causes-of-death.

106 U.S. Centers for Disease Control and Prevention, 'Chronic Disease', October 4, 2024, https://www.cdc.gov/chronic-disease/about/index.html.

107 Mukesh Sharma and P. K. Majumdar, 'Occupational lifestyle diseases: An emerging issue', *Indian journal of occupational and environmental medicine*, 13(3):109-12 (2009), doi:10.4103/0019-5278.58912.

108 Diabetes UK, 'Is There a Cure for Diabetes?', https://www.diabetes.org.uk/diabetes-the-basics/is-there-a-cure.

109 Diabetes UK, 'Research Spotlight – Immunotherapy for Type 1 Diabetes', https://www.diabetes.org.uk/our-research/about-our-research/hot-topics/immunotherapy/what-are-immunotherapies.

110 Type 1 Diabetes The Grand Challenge, https://type1diabetesgrandchallenge.org.uk/.

111 NHS UK, 'What is High Cholesterol?', last reviewed July 13, 2022, https://www.nhs.uk/conditions/high-cholesterol/.

112 American Heart Association, 'Prevention and Treatment of High Cholesterol (Hyperlipidemia)', last reviewed February 19, 2024, https://www.heart.org/en/health-topics/cholesterol/prevention-and-treatment-of-high-cholesterol-hyperlipidemia.

113 World Health Organization, 'Hypertension', March 16, 2023, https://www.who.int/news-room/fact-sheets/detail/hypertension/.

114 U.S. Centers for Disease Prevention and Prevention, 'About Heart Disease', May 15, 2024, https://www.cdc.gov/heart-disease/about/index.html.

115 World Health Organization, 'Cancer', February 3, 2022, https://www.who.int/news-room/fact-sheets/detail/cancer.

116 American Cancer Society, 'Cancer Facts & Figures 2024', *Atlanta: American Cancer Society*, 2024, https://www.cancer.org/content/dam/cancer-org/research/cancer-facts-and-statistics/annual-cancer-facts-and-figures/2024/2024-cancer-facts-and-figures-acs.pdf.

117 U.S. Centers for Disease Control and Prevention, 'Preventing Cancer', October 12, 2023, https://www.cdc.gov/cancer/prevention/?CDC_AAref_Val=https://www.cdc.gov/cancer/dcpc/prevention/index.htm.

118 U.S. Centers for Disease Control and Prevention, 'Treat and Manage High Cholesterol', May 15, 2024, https://www.cdc.gov/cholesterol/

treatment/?CDC_AAref_Val=https://www.cdc.gov/cholesterol/managing-cholesterol.htm.

119 NHS UK, 'High blood pressure', last reviewed July 19, 2024, https://www.nhs.uk/conditions/high-blood-pressure/.

120 World Health Organization, 'Hypertension', March 16, 2023, https://www.who.int/news-room/fact-sheets/detail/hypertension/.

121 World Health Organization, 'Cardiovascular diseases (CVDs)', June 11, 2021, https://www.who.int/news-room/fact-sheets/detail/cardiovascular-diseases-(cvds).

122 World Health Organization, 'Preventing Cancer', https://www.who.int/activities/preventing-cancer.

123 National Institute on Aging, 'Parkinson's Disease: Causes, Symptoms, and Treatments', reviewed April 14, 2022, https://www.nia.nih.gov/health/parkinsons-disease/parkinsons-disease-causes-symptoms-and-treatments.

124 World Health Organization, 'Parkinson disease', August 9, 2023, https://www.who.int/news-room/fact-sheets/detail/parkinson-disease.

125 Lupus Foundation of America, 'What is lupus?', https://www.lupus.org/resources/what-is-lupus.

126 'Health & Cancer Screenings for Women. Which to Prioritize', Harvard Pilgrim Health Care, https://www.harvardpilgrim.org/hapiguide/health-cancer-screenings-for-women-which-to-prioritize/.

127 'Essential Health & Cancer Screenings for Men', Harvard Pilgrim Health Care, https://www.harvardpilgrim.org/hapiguide/essential-health-cancer-screenings-for-men.

128 Penn Heart and Vascular Blog, 'What is a Stress Test?', *Penn Medicine*, July 7, 2022, https://www.pennmedicine.org/updates/blogs/heart-and-vascular-blog/2020/february/what-is-a-stress-test.

129 National Institute of Biomedical Imaging and Bioengineering, 'Computed Topography (CT)', updated June 2022, https://www.nibib.nih.gov/science-education/science-topics/computed-tomography-ct.

130 John Hopkins Medicine, 'Magnetic Resonance Imaging (MRI)', https://www.hopkinsmedicine.org/health/treatment-tests-and-therapies/magnetic-resonance-imaging-mri.

131 The Financial District, 'Redefining Health Care: Mitch Genato', *The Financial District*, October 23, 2023, https://www.thefinancialdistrict. com.ph/post/redefining-healthcare-mitch-genato.

132 IgG Immunoglobin G: This is the most common antibody. It's in blood and other body fluids and protects against bacterial and viral infections.

133 Nutripath, 'Adrenocortex Stress Profile Basic', https://nutripath. com.au/product/cortisol-saliva-test-1001/.

134 Genomind Mental Health Map, 'Frequently Asked Questions', https://mentalhealthmap.com/pages/frequently-asked-questions.

135 MedicubeX, 'eHealth Station™', https://www.medicubex.com/ product.

136 ACT Head Impact Tracker - Northern Sports Insight and Intelligence, https://www.linkedin.com/company/nsii/about/.

137 Dave Asprey, 'What is Biohacking: Infographic', https://daveasprey. com/biohacking-infographic/.

138 Brian Krans, 'What is Leech Therapy?', *Healthline*, updated on April 22, 2017, https://www.healthline.com/health/what-is-leech-therapy/.

139 Jason Jishun Hao and Michele Mittelman, 'Acupuncture: past, present, and future', *Global Advances in Health and Medicine*, 3(4): 6-8 (2014), doi:10.7453/gahmj.2014.042.

140 Sari Harrar, 'Top 5 Medical Breakthroughs of 2023', *AARP*, November 16, 2023, https://www.aarp.org/health/conditions-treatments/info-2023/top-medical-breakthroughs.html.

141 Talia Goldberg, Bhavik Nagda, and Ethan Kurzweil, 'AI escape velocity: A conversation with Ray Kurzweil', *Bessemer Venture Partners*, March 11, 2023, https://www.bvp.com/atlas/ai-escape-velocity-a-conversation-with-ray-kurzweil.

142 Harvard T.H. Chan School of Public Health, 'What's behind "shocking" U.S. life expectancy decline—and what to do about it', April 13, 2023, https://www.hsph.harvard.edu/news/hsph-in-the-news/whats-behind-shocking-u-s-life-expectancy-decline-and-what-to-do-about-it/.

143 SuperAgers, 'Meet the World's Longest Lived', *University of South California*, https://gero.usc.edu/cga/superagers/the-worlds-longest-lived/.

144 Max Planck Institute for Biology of Ageing, 'What do the terms life expectancy, lifespan, longevity and health span mean?', https://www.age.mpg.de/what-do-the-terms-life-expectancy-lifespan-longevity-and-health-span-mean.

145 FNU Sapna et al., 'Advancements in Heart Failure Management: A Comprehensive Narrative Review of Emerging Therapies', *Cureus*, 15(10):e46486 (2023) doi:10.7759/cureus.46486.

146 Institute for Stem Cell & Regenerative Therapy, 'How Does Stem Cell Therapy Work?', *University of Washington*, https://iscrm.uw.edu/how-does-stem-cell-therapy-work/.

147 Kym Burls, 'Tips to Build a Chest Freezer Ice Bath', *Kym Burls*, https://www.kymburls.com/post/tips-to-build-a-chest-freezer-ice-bath.

148 Giovanni Lombardi et al., 'Whole-Body Cryotherapy in Athletes: From Therapy to Stimulation. An Updated Review of the Literature', *Frontiers in Physiology*, 8:258 (May 2, 2017), doi:10.3389/fphys.2017.00258.

149 Kaemmer N. Henderson et al., 'The Cardiometabolic Health Benefits of Sauna Exposure in Individuals with High-Stress Occupations. A Mechanistic Review', *International Journal of Environmental Research and Public Health*, 18(3):1105 (January 27, 2021), doi:10.3390/ijerph18031105.

150 YMCA of Middle Tennessee, 'How the Sauna and Steam Room Can Help Your Health', https://www.ymcamidtn.org/health-and-fitness/articles/how-sauna-and-steam-room-can-help-your-health.

151 Lifeworks, 'Pulsed Electromagnetic Field Therapy (PEMF)', *Lifeworks Wellness Center*, August 5, 2024, https://www.lifeworkswellnesscenter.com/therapies/pulsed-electromagnetic-field-therapy-pemf.html.

152 The Institute for Human Optimization, 'Reverse Oxidative Damage with NanoVi®', https://ifho.org/our-services/nanovi/.

153 Cleveland Clinic, 'Red Light Therapy', last reviewed on January 12, 2021, https://my.clevelandclinic.org/health/articles/22114-red-light-therapy.

154 About the CAROL Bike, https://carolbike.com/.

155 EWOT Team Member, 'EWOT: 6 Effective Benefits- Oxygen Therapy for an Improved Quality of Life', *EWOT*, https://ewot.com/blogs/blog/ewot-6-effective-benefits-oxygen-therapy-for-an-improved-quality-of-life.

156 M. Nathaniel Mead, 'Benefits of sunlight: a bright spot for human health', *Environmental Health Perspectives*, 116(4):A160–7 (2008), doi:10.1289/ehp.116-a160.

157 Jim Robbins, 'Ecopsychology: How Immersion in Nature Benefits Your Health', *Yale Environment 360*, January 9, 2020, https://e360. yale.edu/features/ecopsychology-how-immersion-in-nature-benefits-your-health.